Enjoy Food!!

...and some more myths that still prevent you from doing so

by Pavel Stanishev

This book contains information that is intended to help the readers be better-informed consumers of physical, mental and social health care. It is not intended as a substitute for the medical advice of physicians or doctors. The reader should regularly consult a physician or a doctor in matters relating to his/her health and particularly with respect to any symptoms that may require diagnosis or medical attention.

"Fish and fishermen will always go hand in hand."

author unknown

Table of Contents

Let the myth debunking continue!

I feel the best way to start the first lines of the *"Enjoy Food"* book series sequel, is with one interesting personal story.

I was headed with some friends to the popular Devil's Throat Cave – a truly mystical cave in Bulgaria which I highly recommend that you visit if you have the chance someday.

So, we were in the car, enjoying nature around and having all sorts of discussions. Of course, we touched upon some of my favorite topics – nutrition, sport, and diets.

We talked about how people still pay a lot of money for template eating plans from known and unknown doctors and nutritionists, how they stuff themselves with a bunch of supplements and never achieve any lasting and steady results. We talked about how certain types of food are so overhyped and how others are considered extremely unhealthy. We also chatted about how masses of people are obsessed with "healthy" and "balanced" eating but how different diets always make them suffer physically, mentally, and socially.

And as we were already wrapping up the debate, I suddenly ended up stating the following:

"Fish and fishermen will always go hand in hand".

The moment I heard myself saying that I was already imagining including it as a quote in the sequel of the "Enjoy Food" book series. But, of course, I had to look that up on the Internet and see who the author of these words was.

To my surprise, I didn't find any information. Well, that's kind of bizarre, isn't it? I quoted something popular, I was sure about that... but I never actually found a track of it anywhere.

So, if anyone knows who the father of those so true words was, please look me up in the social networks and share that to me - I promise that I'll make the necessary corrections immediately.

And yet, in the context of dieting and eating, these words describe pretty well that until we start seeing the whole picture and until we start looking for more reliable and evidence-based information on what the true healthy eating actually is, all the marketers, dishonest (or simply unaware) fitness instructors, and food industry, in general, will continue taking advantage of our lack of knowledge, naivety and false illusions.

If you've already read the first book of the series, you'd know a little bit more about what needs to raise your concerns and what not when it comes to sugar, detox, salt, saturated fats, gluten, GMO, organic foods, hormones in animal products, processed foods, etc. – yes, without a doubt, the negative beliefs related to them are among the most popular myths that make us see some of the foods as bad and unhealthy.

But you don't think that these are the only ones, do you?...

Well, to our great misfortunate – yes, these aren't the only nutrition myths at all.

But, luckily, there are papers like the one you're reading that are written with the sole purpose of making you a bit more aware and look at things from a different perspective, based on critical thinking and logic, but mostly – on some other dozens of scientific case studies, causes, meta-analysis, reviews, and conclusions.

And I strongly believe that all the information we'll review in the next pages will help you learn how to better avoid the numerous "fishermen's hooks" in the future.

Without any further announcements – as the title of the chapter clearly says, let the food myth debunking go on!

The ultimate diet – myth or... reality

When I think about it, I realize that I meet new people relatively often. Most of the times, we end up chatting about diets, we discuss cooking, recipes, eating habits, food preferences, nutrition myths, and truths. Yet, it seems that the most common question that they ask me is usually something similar to *"Well, then, tell me which is the best diet to lose weight!"*

Keto diet, gluten-free diet, 90-day diet, DASH diet, detox diet, low-fat diet, low-carb diet, Mediterranean diet, Moon diet, apple diet, IIFYM, zodiac diet, blood type-based diet, paleo diet...

Yes, the list of diets is truly endless.

Many people don't really think about that, but the simple truth is that each one of them is based on the very same principle – knowingly or not, every popular diet aims to put us in an *energy deficit*. As we know, and as it has been scientifically proven many times, this is the *most* important factor for losing weight (and I say "weight" and not "fats" on purpose). And yes, any of these diets could work for us – yet, we have the most important condition met – to consume less energy than the one we use.

Diet	How it works?	What does it lead to?
Keto	Low carb, high fat & protein	Caloric deficit
Paleo	Eat no processed foods	Caloric deficit
IIFYM	Track macros and calories	Caloric deficit
Apple diet	Eat apples only	Caloric deficit

BUT! Problems always start *after* our diet ends. If we manage to reach that end of it at all... And these problems are very similar, no matter the diet's name.

Before we proceed, I'd like to point out that I'd avoid as much as possible the use of scientific literature in this a bit longer chapter. Even though it'd support all the statements we make, I do believe that in the context of the topic, it'd be enough to just use some critical and logical thinking.

Popular diets are temporary

Unfortunately, the great majority of the diets that we hear and read about everywhere, are *time-oriented* – in other words, they have been created to last only for a *limited* period. They have an existing end date. And past that date, they're simply... over. We can easily get to that characteristic by simply asking questions like "*Are you on a diet now?*", "*How long do you have to follow that diet?*" and so on.

Let's take the keto diet, for instance. It has led to excellent results with millions of people who had followed it, but does this mean that all these people could live their whole lives following its rules and hard restrictions? Or can people "detox" themselves all the time simply because this type of diet advises so? And how could you possibly be on the 90-day diet till the end of your days if the very *name* of the diet suggests that it's valid for 90 days only?

Okay, yes, there could be some who somehow manage to turn the temporary diets into a permanent lifestyle but let's not split hairs and just concentrate on the common rule and not on the rare exceptions.

So, there is a head-on collision with the first big issue - namely, the well-known diets are often *temporary*.

And temporary solutions lead only to temporary results. Yes, if we need an eating plan to help us get in some old suit for an important event in two weeks, then most of the diets could do us a very nice job. However, if we're extremely overweight and there is a serious risk to our physical health (which often is related to some mental load, too) then is this 90-day diet the best choice for us? This is just a rhetorical question.

Remember, diets should be *sustainable*! The best diet for you is the one that you'd be able to follow in the *long* term. The best diet for you leads to a *permanent* change in your eating habits. And the best diet does *not* have a duration. If you cannot keep following the diet even after you've achieved the desired results, then this diet is simply not fit for you.

Popular diets lack individualism

Now we get to the second huge issue – it's that almost none of the popular diets are based on the principle of *individualism*.

Yet, if we think about it, each one of us is a unique biological entity and has different daily routines, habits, hobbies, personal preferences and so on.

For example, I don't like pumpkin. I also don't like olives. And I feel most comfortable when I have 3-4 meals a day. And often I don't feel hungry in the mornings. These are just a few of my personal characteristics that come to my mind as a start, without even having any deep thoughts on that. And having in mind these only characteristics, how many diets would fit in my lifestyle? Truth is that the list would shorten very quickly.

So, well, I don't like pumpkin and olives, then I wouldn't eat them. Every diet could work around that. But what should I do if the diet that I've chosen, states that I have to eat 5-6-7 times a day? I wouldn't feel comfortable at all - as I said, I prefer having large meals 3-4 times a day. How many diets would satisfy that "whim" of mine?

And what about the fact that I'm rarely hungry in the morning? But when I look at the "rules" of the newest, most trending diet – it clearly says that in the mornings I *must* eat this and that. Okay, but I simply don't want to eat at that time of the day! It turns out that I have to force-feed myself...

And what would happen if we add a few similar factors from our daily routine or some other 5-6 eating preferences? Yes, it gets complicated. A lot.

Truth is that everyone wants a universal answer, a template, a scheme or an hourly breakdown of the meals. For everyone's regret, however, so far, there is not a single diet that could work for *all* of us.

Remember, diets should be *personalized*! They have to fit your daily routine and your personal eating preferences.

Okay, so far we've reviewed how the popular diets are often time-oriented and even more often – not individualized. These are indeed two big issues. But there's a third one as well – it's that most of those diets are way too *restrictive*.

Popular diets are way too restrictive

You have to agree that there is no way to keep following a diet that turns our life into a nightmare – it tortures us, terrorizes us and makes us think only about the forbidden yummies.

Yes, in theory, if we just stop eating foods like pizza and chocolate, it'd be the healthiest possible choice.

Stop consuming them once and for all!

Till the end of our days!

But let's be completely honest, how many would resist eating chocolate and pizza till the very end of their lives? This is yet another rhetorical question.

It's true, from a physical point of view, pizza and chocolate aren't needed in our menu at all. I agree. But the complete restriction of these foods would most definitely influence negatively both our *mental* health and *social* life.

Can you imagine what the effect would be if we forbid someone who loves having just a single block of chocolate every other day from eating chocolate at all? Very often the first thing that happens when we restrict a certain food is to have an even stronger desire to eat *exactly* that type of food. That's why the long time spent without chocolate or pizza often leads to unstoppable binge eating precisely with... chocolate or pizza.

And let's be honest, from time to time it happens to every one of us to overeat. When we have the "hard restriction mode" turned on for a long period, however, these episodes are very likely to happen more often and the overeating itself gets far more serious – it turns into out-of-control binge eating.

For that reason, when we allow ourselves certain types of foods in minor quantities in our daily diet, these episodes are expected to be more sporadic or at least – they wouldn't be that extreme. That's why being *flexible* with the food products we consume is of big importance.

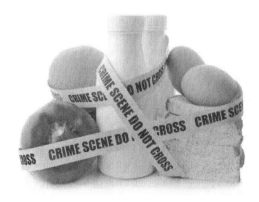

Remember, diets should *not* be *too* restrictive! They should *not* torture us and make us to only think about all the "forbidden" foods. Exactly these "forbidden" foods have a quite significant place in a really good diet as their consumption from time to time could help us in keeping better track of the diet we follow.

It's much better if we're 80% accurate in our diet 80% of the time rather than being 100% accurate but in just 50% of the time, don't you think?

How do ALL popular diets work?

And in order not to be vague in my statements (as we mentioned the phrase "most popular diets" several times now), it'd be a good idea to see how these popular diets actually work and then logically seek the three big issues we've talked about: time-orientation, lack of individualism and excessive restrictiveness.

As said at the beginning of the chapter, every diet is based on putting our bodies in a caloric deficit mode. This deficit works by reducing the intake of one (or more) of the three food macronutrients: *carbohydrates, fats,* and *proteins.*

This immediately could lead us to the thought that the number of possible combinations between the nutrients is not that large. That's the reason why diets are most commonly based on one of the three basic principles:

- Fewer carbohydrates and more fats
- Fewer carbohydrates and more proteins
- More carbohydrates and fewer fats

Atkins/keto/low-carb diets

The first and the second principle serve as a basic idea for most of the well-known diets, including the Atkins diet and the incredibly famous keto diet.

Diets of that kind encourage the intake of foods rich in proteins and fats. This means that you'd have a wide variety of animal products – meat, dairy, eggs, and fish. The only macronutrient that is under strict monitoring is the carbohydrates.

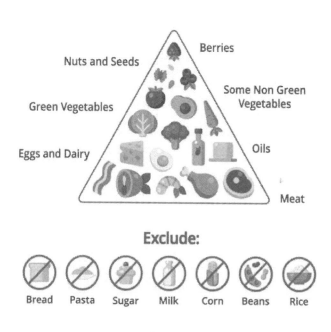

Keto food pyramid
Source: theketobroad.com

At first, it might seem pretty easy to follow these rules, but, in practice, it's far from true - at least for a great part of the people who have tried and failed the diet.

Because those who aren't familiar with Atkins or keto would assume that the carbs restriction means a restriction only on the "bad" foods – donuts, chocolate, and croissants. Reality is that apart from them, the consumption of many fruits and even a large portion of the vegetables is extremely prohibited. The purpose of this is to reduce the carbs to the drastic levels of about 50 grams (or even less) per day.

Just to help you picture this – this is approximately the number of carbs in a *single* large banana.[1]

Of course, here is the place to mention the so-called *"ketosis"* – a metabolic process that occurs when the body begins to burn fat for energy because it doesn't have enough carbohydrates to use. During this process, the liver produces chemicals called *ketones*. And the keto diet aims to induce ketosis in order to burn more fat.

But let's not go off-topic and stick to the main point.

In short, are these diets restrictive? Definitely yes – they're *extremely* restrictive.

For example, as a great fan of any fruit, rice, and potatoes, I'd find it very hard to follow a diet that eliminates the consumption of these foods in the long run. Here we mention again the principle of individualism – I like carbs and I love consuming them. Yes, I could restrict their intake to some level, but no way I can practically eliminate them. These types of diets are far away from me and my daily routine and preferences, I find them way too strenuous and restrictive.

And this applies not only for me but for millions of people out there - perhaps you, too?

Of course, millions have seen and felt great results from the low-carb diets, and they have their right to defend them. But let's not go to extremes and proclaim them for the best diets.

Because they are not.

Such a low intake of carbohydrates often leads to stomach disorders, dehydration, fatigue, nausea, vomiting, lack of motivation and other concerning symptoms. And if we just think for a second, with this type of diet, the quantity of the fruit and vegetables that are consumed is quite small which, on the other hand, means lower intake of vitamins and minerals.

And this, on its own, is another risk factor to our health.

Low-fat diets

There are quite a few diets that follow the opposite principle – high consumption of carbohydrates with a hard restriction on the intake of fats.

In other words – a lot of fruits, vegetables, and even pasta. Proteins are in moderate quantities but yet the meat should not be fatty, and the dairy products should be skimmed. Fish isn't recommended here and products such as butter, yolks, olive oil and vegetable oil are on the verge of being "prohibited".

Even though at first it might seem good that the diet allows us to eat more carbs, most people abuse that and eat far too much bread and pasta, for instance. Indeed, these foods taste awesome, but they also have a low quantity of fibers and their macronutrient profile is far from impressive, as well.

And yet, it shouldn't be a surprise when we say that the *real* problem of the diets of that kind is rooted in the low intake of fats. As they're a key component for the taste qualities of the food, for many people eating food without any fats would mean only one simple thing – *tasteless* food.

And would it be possible for us to keep following a diet that is based on food that doesn't taste good for us? No, of course not.

And I don't even want to go in more detail about how important dietary fats are for our health and how following such a diet goes hand in hand with the high risk of not taking enough fatty acids – the ones that our bodies *cannot* synthesize on their own.

Some not-so-popular forms of the low-fat diets even restrict to a high extent the intake of proteins, as well. That, along with the low intake of fats, could simply mean insufficient intake of fat-soluble vitamins.

To summarize what we've said so far – low-carb diets are highly restrictive, and they restrain us from eating extremely important dietary products, such as fruits and vegetables. And because of those restrictions, for most people, following these diets over a long period is questionable.

The situation with low-fat diets is almost identical – not only they test our will in the long run, but they could also even be potentially dangerous because of the low intake of nutrients that are essential for our health.

Surely, the list of diets that are based on low-carb or low-fat meals is the longest, but this doesn't mean that they're the only ones available.

One-food-only diets

There are quite a few eating plans which impose the consumption of only one type of food – for example, the apple "diet". There are also these, let's say, more "liberal" ones that allow you to choose what to eat – only bananas, only potatoes or only oranges. Often the rule is quite simple – when you feel hungry, consume only the food that you have chosen and nothing else.

As you might have probably guessed by now – such way of is not healthy at all, it's highly unbalanced and even foolish.

I wouldn't go any further but will only say that such "diets" stimulate the development of bad eating habits and even – eating disorders.

Diets based on blood type, moon phase, zodiac etc.

The situation with all the fad diets that are based on fabricated information about the physiology and metabolism of our bodies is quite similar.

There are quite a few people who believe that blood type, moon phases or zodiac signs are the factors that determine the best way of how we should be dieting.

Blood Type	Characteristics	Best Foods	Worst Foods	Foods that Aid this Blood Type the Best
Type O	Known to have strong immune and digestive systems. Type Os also have efficient metabolisms and are naturally hardy against illnesses.	High protein foods (lean meat and fish), legumes, pulses, soy, nuts (cashews, pecans, all-natural peanut butter), yellow & red vegetables and fruits	Wheat, corn, kidney beans, navy beans, lentils, cabbage, brussels sprouts, cauliflower	Kelp, seafood, salt, liver, red meat, kale, spinach and broccoli
Type A	Those with type A blood can adapt well to dietary and environmental changes. They generally have a good immune system, and are able to metabolize nutrients easily.	Type A's will best benefit from a vegetarian diet that includes a wide array of vegetables, as well as tofu, seafood, grains, beans, legumes and fruit	Most types of meat, dairy, kidney beans, lima beans, wheat	Vegetable oil, soy-based foods, vegetables and fruits, particularly pineapple.
Type B	Have strong immune systems; can adapt readily to dietary and environmental changes; known to have balanced nervous systems	Meat (no chicken), dairy, grains, beans, legumes, vegetables and fruit.	Corn, lentils, peanuts, sesame seeds, buckwheat and wheat	Dark leafy greens, eggs, venison, liver, licorice and tea
Type AB	Type ABs have extremely efficient tolerant immune systems. They are technically a combination of the benefits of both A and B blood types.	Lean meat (in moderation), seafood, dairy, tofu, beans, legumes, grains, vegetables and fruit	Red meat, kidney beans, lima beans, seeds, corn and buckwheat	Tofu, seafood, dairy, greens, kelp, seaweed (nori), and pineapple

Blood type diet is a F-A-D diet

There are also beliefs that the weight that we put on is mainly due to a liver malfunctioning as it gets "clogged" with toxins. And this is how all the detox diets were born (*more about the detox topic is to be found in the first book of the "Enjoy Food" series*).

Such "diets" aren't balanced even from a nutritional point of view. They almost always lack vital amino acids, vitamins, fatty acids, fibers and so on. And this has many hidden risks to our health.

Yet another problem that only a few of us actually think about, is that the absurd points of view that are in the basis of those "diets" actually replace the real, evidence-based theories of dietology and nutritionism. As a result, people get an unreal and confusing vision of what healthy eating should really be.

Flexible diet (IIFYM)

In recent years, the IIFYM protocol (*If It Fits Your Macros*) has gained in popularity. It's also known as the "*flexible diet*".

The idea of that type of eating is for everyone to determine their individual caloric and macronutrient intake that would lead them to a caloric deficit (or caloric surplus in case weight gaining is the aim) and to be aware of what they eat and more importantly – in what *quantities*.

In general, the rule is that we can include *any* type of food on our menu as long as we don't exceed the set target of calories and macronutrients.

Contrary to most popular diets, this one almost lacks restrictiveness – yes, we have to take no more than X calories per day, but we have the freedom to choose from what food sources they'd come. We can practically have different dishes every day and even with every meal. In this way, we can personalize our dieting to the tiniest detail possible.

What a great advantage!

Just think about what does it mean to have personalization and reasonable restrictiveness when it comes to dieting? It means that we can follow the diet for a long time and achieve long-lasting results with it!

Now probably you'd ask yourselves if we've found the ultimate diet, right?

Unfortunately, this is not exactly the case...

Even though I'm a great supporter of IIFYM, I cannot admit that it might have a slew of hidden drawbacks to some people.

First, to be 100% sure that you correctly follow the flexible diet, you need to *measure* the quantity of every food that you eat. This means that you have to weigh *everything* on the kitchen scales and to enter the details of it in a mobile app. Every single time. Every single day.

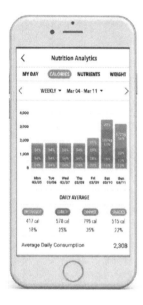

And this activity, especially at the beginning, really takes a lot of effort and time.

Okay, let's say that we (somehow) have enough time and this is not a problem for us. But what happens when we decide to go out with friends or family to have some dinner? We can do no more but only try to guess the weight of the products used in the meals on the menu.

Moreover, we cannot be even sure whether the total weight stated in the menu is correct.

The second drawback of IIFYM is that it quite often has the potential to "encourage" people to include foods with little to none micronutrients in their eating plan just because the calories allow such flexibility.

After all, the idea of following whichever diet, in general, is to be *healthy* – it'd be hard to achieve that if the main foods that we eat are chocolate, ice-cream, spaghetti, pizza, bread and many others of that kind, even if they fit our macros.

Yes, they could hit the *macros*, but they wouldn't hit the *micros*.

Despite its shortcomings, the flexible diet helped for the great results for millions of people all over the world. And yet, following that plan of eating is a *skill* which, if you have the will to develop, could help you turn this plan into a part of your life.

Into a lifestyle.

Building YOUR OWN diet – the pillars

Okay, what kind of diet should we follow then?

If what we claim is true (and namely, that the ultimate diet that could work for everyone doesn't exist – it's a myth), then how can we find the correct way of eating?

The good news is that yet there are a few simple rules and conditions which, when balanced, could help you create the best, the most efficient and easy to follow personalized diet – the one that is only for *you*.

We've already discussed why the eating plan should be *individualized* according to your preferences and daily round, why it shouldn't be too *restrictive* and why we need to turn it into a lifestyle that would cost us *minimal* efforts to achieve *steady* results.

Now, let's review, what I call the "four pillars" of the true diet – these are rules which we should never make a compromise with.

1st pillar – energy deficit

First of all – make sure that you're really in a caloric deficit.

You might eat only the perfect "superfoods" (*we'll talk about them later*) and to obtain all the vitamins and minerals, but if you consume *more* energy than the one you burn, you'd simply *not* lose weight!

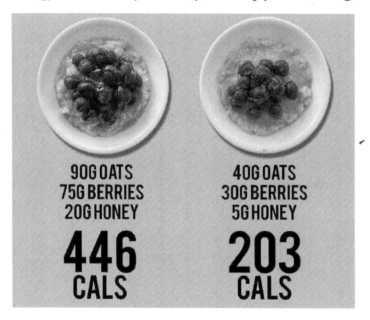

90G OATS
75G BERRIES
20G HONEY
446
CALS

40G OATS
30G BERRIES
5G HONEY
203
CALS

Spot the difference - portion control is crucial

If needed, you can try the flexible diet out for a couple of weeks just to understand at what calories you slowly start losing weight.

2ⁿᵈ pillar – muscle mass

The next rule, unfortunately, is usually neglected by a lot of people. It seems to be considered not that important but, in fact, it's SO important. That's why I'm willing to pay a little bit more attention to it.

Remember, the true diet should help you maintaining (and even improving) your *muscle mass*. After all, we follow diets and eat healthily in the name of better health and better appearance, don't we? Let me then explain to you why maintaining your muscle mass is a fundamental condition to achieve all of that.

Probably there were times when you were thinking something similar to: *"I want to get rid of this damn fat, I don't care about my muscle mass at all, I don't want big muscles - I just want to lose the ugly fat!"* Even if you haven't thought this yourself, I'm pretty sure that you've at least heard someone else grumble about it.

Truth is that there are a few major reasons that should make you think twice about preserving and improving your muscle mass.

First, muscles are the ones that give us *shape*. No matter how many fats and kilos you lose, if you don't have enough muscle mass, you'd never have a good-looking figure. And this is valid for both men *and* women. Here I need to turn to the ladies with the consolation that building muscle mass is an extremely hard and slow process, especially for you. That's why you don't have to be afraid of doing sport, it can only be one of your best friends and an ally in the fight for the well-sculpted body.

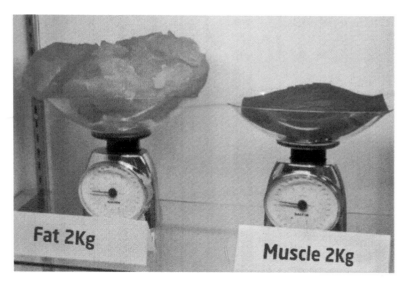

Think FAT loss, not WEIGHT loss
Source: zumub.com

Second – our bodies require much more *energy* maintaining the muscle mass than maintaining the fats.

In contrast to fats, muscle mass is an *active* tissue - muscles work even when we're in rest. In practice, every movement, even the unconscious one, would be impossible without the activation of a given muscle. And the quantity of muscle mass we have has a greater influence on the calories that we burn when we are in *rest*.

Let me give you this example – if we have a bit bigger and stronger muscles, we'd burn more fats in any other moment – even when we're just lying on the sofa, when we're at the office, while we do sports and even when we sleep. If you think about it, this means that we'll burn the same amount of fats while we eat more food. This, on the other hand, would lead to less hunger, longer-lasting diet, and much better results.

3rd pillar – protein

And there is no way to keep and build muscles in our bodies if we don't take enough *protein*. Therefore, the next rule for a perfect diet is related exactly to the intake of protein.

There are many, many scientific works proving that a diet rich in protein might have a lot of positive effects.

For example, when under the same circumstances, people who take more protein lose similar weight, but by burning *more* fat mass and *less* muscle mass.[2][3] And this translates into better body composition, which means better look, which means better confidence, which means more happiness.

Besides, it's been proven that protein *satiates more* compared with the other two macronutrients – carbohydrates and fats.[4] And as we can guess, *hunger* is the main *enemy* in the fight with weight. And the hungrier we get, the greater the possibility to binge eat is.

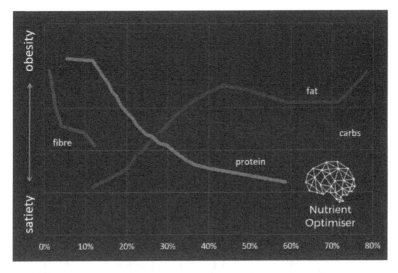

More protein consumption means less hunger
Source: optimisingnutrition.com

And last but not least, when compared again with fats and carbohydrates, protein has the highest *thermic effect of food* (TEF).

In brief, this is a parameter that indicates what percentage of the caloricity of a given food is needed for its intake and absorption.

The scientific works showed that usually 25-30% of the calorie value of protein is needed for its absorption. Just for comparison, the percentage of the carbs is 6-8% and one of the fats is even lower – 2-3%.[5][6]

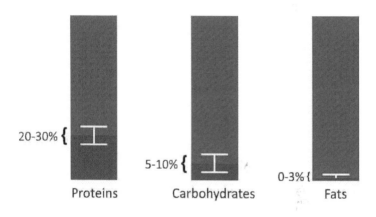

In short, protein is awesome

Of course, it wouldn't be a good idea to go in the opposite direction and start eating way too much protein. Indeed, the high intake of protein is safe except with people with prominent kidney diseases, but this doesn't mean that more protein is for the better. When we're in a huge caloric deficit, the excessive amount of protein doesn't have any additional contribution but is at the expense of fats and carbs.

This would simply destroy the balance of the diet and would also result in fewer meal options for us to choose from.

4th pillar – time

And now, we reached the last fundamental pillar – *stop looking for quick solutions*!

If you simply want to play the '*lose weight-gain weight*' game, then the common short-term diets would be very useful to you... But if you do want to completely change the way you look, to be in your best shape and to feel better in your skin for the years to come, you need to look for a solution in the long run.

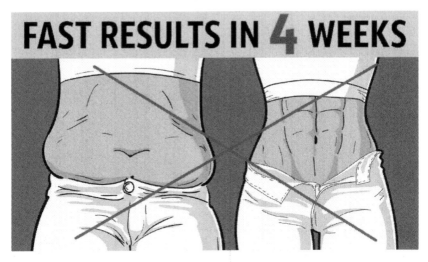

Fast results for fast failures

And please don't think only about what and how much of it you eat, just pay attention to sports and physical *activity* too.

Training is an integral part of having a good body, so don't give up on it. You should find an activity that is interesting for you and that makes you happy and spend at least an hour a few times a week doing it and very soon you'd feel an incredible difference.

You already know that but it's always a good reminder - the more you try to avoid the sedentary lifestyle, the better!

And when you combine the sufficient activity and the good eating plan (based on the rules mentioned above) you'd not only once and for all achieve the desired results but would also learn to fight with challenges and *not* give up when you are faced with them.

Choose the long run – it's hard and thorny, but it strengthens and teaches how to fight, how to be disciplined and how to be persevering – all this will affect favorably not only the appearance but also the strength of your *character.*

And who wouldn't like being considered to have a healthy mind in a healthy body?

The big picture

To finalize, let's just summarize the most important characteristics of the ultimate diet – the one that doesn't have a specific name:

- The ultimate diet does *not* last for a certain period. It develops good eating *habits* and changes our daily routine for the better.
- The ultimate diet is *individualized* according to our preferences and lifestyle.
- The ultimate diet is *not too restrictive* but yet it puts us in a caloric *deficit.*
- The ultimate diet does not make us feel strong *hunger.*
- The ultimate diet is rich in *protein* and encourages us to do more sports and to have a more *active* lifestyle.
- The ultimate diet results in slow but *long-lasting* results.

And, of course, as the title of the book suggests:

- The ultimate diet must combine *all* of the above-mentioned points and bring *pleasure* to the whole process

Indeed, the best diets for which you constantly hear and read about are only a myth for most of us. That's why you simply need to make sure that you have a well-balanced choice of food, you do sports, you're physically active – but most importantly, you learn to enjoy all of that!

Aspartame and some non-artificial facts

In the long gone 1965, in an attempt to create a new medicine against ulcer, the chemist James Schlatter discovered something that shook the foundations of the food industry and dietology in the next decades.

The substance he discovered had great characteristics – it was 200 times *sweeter* than sugar and practically had *no* calories! The name of that substance - *aspartame*.

In the next more than 50 years after the discovery of aspartame, its incredible sweetness, use, and safety will continue raising unabated arguments and discussions among the people.

We've all heard of aspartame. We also know what it is – an *artificial* sweetener that is used in thousands of products in the world – fizzy (diet) drinks, chewing gums, dessert bars, and many others.

And millions indeed consume these products so that they could allow themselves the tasty pleasures in question without exceeding their calorie intake and without gaining weight.

But the amount of people who frankly demonize the sweetener and swear in its negative effect on our health is quite considerable as well. They also spread conspiracies if the whole truth about aspartame has been shared with us at all and if it has been kept a secret because of industrial, marketing, and financial reasons.

In this chapter, we'll leave the conspiracy theories behind along with what we see on TV, magazines and the Internet. Yet, if we want to have truly objective information for whatever statement, it'd be reasonable to turn to science, not to Fox News, Cosmopolitan or Facebook, wouldn't it?

What is aspartame?

Those of you who have sharp eyes probably have noticed that it was emphasized on the fact that aspartame is an *artificial* sweetener. And that single word started the first attacks on the substance – *"Why do you praise the artificial sweeteners so much, they're pure chemical poison to your body!"*

Indeed, artificial sweeteners are chemical production... But so does sugar. Strawberries are chemistry, avocados are chemistry, water is chemistry, and the air is chemistry. So what?

In fact, if you want to understand in detail my opinion about the "it's chemistry" type of accusations, I encourage you to read the "It's ALL Chemistry!" chapter from the first book of the *"Enjoy Food"* series.

That's why I'd continue and not repeat the same statements here.

The more important thing is not if aspartame is chemistry, but what *kind* of chemistry it is. What we know from the numerous lab tests and analyses is that we can digest it easily and thoroughly. In other words, the substance could be found in our body just for a short time and neither it nor any of its components could be accumulated in our body.[7]

It's of significant importance to understand what is left in our bodies after the decomposition of aspartame – namely, 50% *phenylalanine*, 40% *aspartic acid*, and 10% *methanol*.[8] All three substances are also found in many other foods and we'll briefly review them one by one.

Aspartic acid   **Phenylalanine**

Methanol

This is what aspartame looks like from a chemical point of view.

Phenylalanine

Okay, let's see what we need to know about *phenylalanine* – this is an essential amino acid which means that our body can only supply it from food.

Phenylalanine is often found naturally in many foods that contain protein – all types of meat, dairy and wheat products.

In a standard can of a diet soft drink, we can find around 125 mg aspartame[9] which means that phenylalanine is slightly above 60 mg (since we said it's roughly 50% of the sweetener).

Now, let's just compare the approximate amount of 60 mg which could be found in that single can with a couple of other foods that also contain phenylalanine[10]:

- 100 grams of parmesan cheese contain 1922 mg (above 30 times more)

- 100 grams of pumpkin seeds contain 1733 mg (approximately 28 times more)
- 100 grams of lean roasted beef contain 1464 mg (almost 24 times more)
- 100 grams of cooked chicken breasts contain 1294 mg (above 20 times more)
- 100 grams of cooked tuna fist contains 1101 mg (above 17 times more)
- A SINGLE egg contains 340 mg (almost 6 times more)

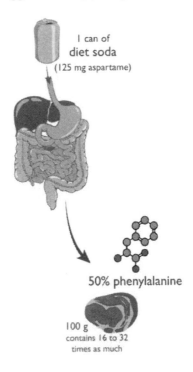

Source: mennohenselmans.com

And that's not all – in order to complete the whole point of that comparison, here we need to see what the acceptable daily intake (ADI) of aspartame is.

According to the US Food and Drug Administration (FDA), an intake in the measurement of up to 50 mg/kg per day is safe for human consumption.[11]

The European Food Safety Authority (EFSA) recommends a little bit lower, but yet similar number – 40 mg/kg.[12]

The same quantity is also recommended by the World Health Organization (WHO).[13]

Organization	Aspartame ADI
US Food and Drug Administration (FDA)	50 mg/kg
European Safety Authority (EFSA)	40 mg/kg
World Health Organization (WHO)	40 mg/kg

You can go through the information provided by dozens of other health and science organizations and you'll see that they're all unanimous in the amounts of safe daily intake of aspartame.

Having said that, let's see one simple hypothetic example – with 40 mg/kg of acceptable daily intake and the 125 mg of aspartame that are found in a diet coke can, we can easily do some math and see that a 50-kilogram woman could safely consume *up to 16 cans* of the drink without any health risks.

I repeat – *sixteen* cans! That is more than *5 liters* of coke! Per day! And that's the daily intake of a 50-kilogram person - for the heavier ones, the intake would be even higher. It wouldn't be a surprise if I say that there are only a few people that can barely reach these quantities.[14]

And now, let's jump back to phenylalanine.

Truth is that it's perfectly safe (when consumed reasonably, of course) for most of us.

Unfortunately, some people suffer from the rare genetic disease called *phenylketonuria* (PKU) where the intake of the amino acid is dangerous as it might accumulate in the body and cause severe brain damages. That's why all the products (including the medications) that contain aspartame, have to be avoided by those people. And this is the reason why these products also have a label stating: *"Contains Phenylalanine"*.

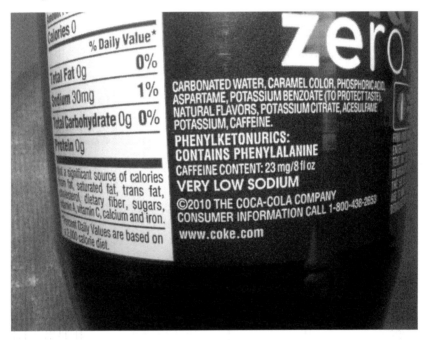

For some, phenylalanine could be dangerous
Source: dyediet.com

Still, the good news is that the reported incidence of PKU from newborn screening programs ranges from one in 13 500 to 19 000 newborns in the United States.[15]

Aspartic acid

After phenylalanine, let's pay some attention to the second amino acid that is found in our bodies after the aspartame decomposition – 40% of it breaks into *aspartic acid*.

In contrast to phenylalanine, aspartic acid is nonessential. In other words, our body cells can produce that amino acid, which is why we don't need to supply it from the food.

Still, this is hard to follow as the substance could be found in many other food products – all types of meat, eggs, fish, nuts, seeds, leafy greens, fruits, vegetables, etc.

Similar to phenylalanine, the content of aspartic acid in a can of diet coke is many times less than in 100 grams of any other product that naturally contains it.

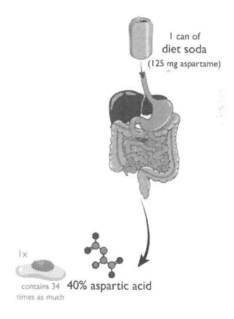

I can of
diet soda
(125 mg aspartame)

Ix
contains 34 **40% aspartic acid**
times as much

Source: mennohenselmans.com

Methanol

The third component of aspartame, which is barely 10% of it, is *methanol* - the substance that lays in the majority of the accusations against the artificial sweetener.

Methanol is a type of alcohol which in certain (of course, extremely high) doses could be poisonous and even cancerogenic (in other words – increasing the risk of cancer development).

However, as we know – the dose makes the poison. Truth is that aspartame contains so insignificant amounts of methanol, that even a glass of tomato juice has 6 times *more* methanol than the one in a can of diet coke.

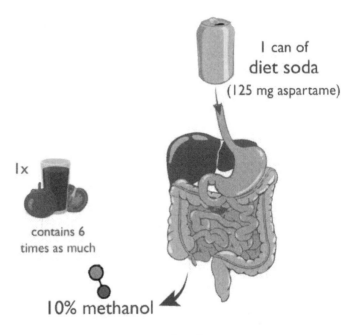

I can of
diet soda
(125 mg aspartame)

1x

contains 6
times as much

10% methanol

Source: mennohenselmans.com

Besides, the daily toxicological reference dose of methanol is 0.5 mg/kg.[16] This means that the woman from the previous example weighted at 50 kilograms can take up to 25 mg of methanol daily with a very low risk of any issues.

Let's also recall that a can of diet coke has about 125 mg of aspartame – simple math shows that the amount of methanol is just around 1.25 mg per can. This means that the woman from the example could potentially drink up to *20 cans* of diet soft drinks... per day!

Nevertheless, methanol (and respectively, aspartame) has been demonized by the mass of people and has been directly related to many insidious health issues.

For example, it's been widely believed that it can cause blindness. However, the European Food Safety Authority (EFSA) once again declared that the methanol delivered by aspartame is in such insignificant quantities that these fears are simply unjustified.[17]

And let's remind again that methanol from aspartame cannot be accumulated in our body, so respectively it's almost impossible for it to reach any dangerous levels, even if we decide to go to extremes with the sugar-free drinks, for some reason.

Aspartame and headache

Yet, this is only the beginning – aspartame is associated with so many more kinds of evil. Headache, for example.

Thousands of people swear they have a really strong headache shortly after consuming a product that contains the sweetener. Even though science literature doesn't support that accusation explicitly, social networks, TV, and magazines blare it forth.

There are quite a few researches that conclude that there is no difference in the headache occurrence of people who take aspartame and people who don't.[18] [19] [20]

Unfortunately, that is still not enough to make the truth stronger than the myth.

Aspartame and muscle/bone pain

Very often we can hear or read that aspartame significantly complicates the condition of people who suffer from *fibromyalgia* (a medical condition characterized by strong pain in muscles and bones).

As you can guess, however, this should also be classified as a "myth".

For instance, in 2014, one pretty eye-opening research was held on 72 women. They were divided into two groups and one of them was forbidden to consume aspartame-containing products.

Nevertheless, no difference in the power of the fibromyalgia pains has been established – the lack of aspartame consumption in one of the groups didn't lead to symptoms improvement, and vice versa – taking aspartame over a long period didn't lead to change for the worse in the other group of women.[21]

Aspartame and epilepsy

Aspartame doesn't lead to epileptic fits increase too. Even though quite a few people believe otherwise.

Only a few pieces of research on that subject have been held but their results are all definitive.

One of them, for instance, was held on 10 kids with epilepsy who were divided into two groups - the first group consumed aspartame and the second one – not. The research period was two weeks. The results showed no differences which could make the scientists believe that aspartame and the epileptic fits are somehow related.[22]

The conclusions made from another research are identical – in that case, 18 people were under supervision, and part of them took aspartame in tablets while the others took placebo tablets – nothing that could raise concerns was noticed.[23]

Aspartame and cancer

However, the most widespread and hard to break through are the beliefs that aspartame can directly cause cancer.

Interestingly, this fear is relatively new.

It started back in 2005 when Italian scientists from the Ramazzini Institute found out that the high intake of the artificial sweetener could increase the risk of leukemia in *rats*.[24]

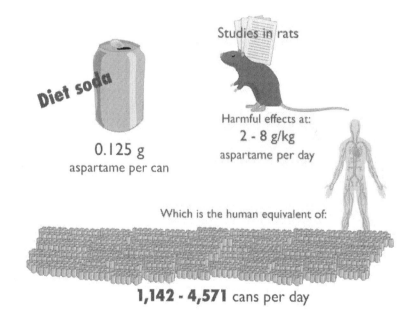

Studies in rats

Diet soda

0.125 g
aspartame per can

Harmful effects at:
2 - 8 g/kg
aspartame per day

Which is the human equivalent of:

1,142 - 4,571 cans per day

Source: mennohenselmans.com

Even though it was clearly and broadly stated that the study was conducted on animals, human psychology instantly unleashed intense suspiciousness and anxiety.

Affected by the newly discovered threat, the American Food and Drug Administration (FDA) decided to study in detail the methodology of that study. They established some imperfections in the design and not a few discrepancies in the way of conducting the research.[25]

That's why, in the same year, the National Cancer Institute (NCI) repeated the whole study using better methods (a larger group of test rats that were separated in different groups; tests conducted for a longer period and so on). And they didn't find any presence of cancer growths or any cancer-related risks.[26]

The European Food Safety Authority (EFSA) also decided to review the results reached by the Ramazzini Institute and similarly to the National Cancer Institute, they also found some discrepancies in the conclusions of the Italian scientists – lack of any relation between the tumors found in rats and the aspartame treatment, lack of conclusion in terms of substance consumption by humans, lack of data in terms of the proportion dosage and response to that dosage, and many others. As a result, they published again their statement that aspartame safety to humans had been incorrectly doubted and the substance remains safe for human consumption on the condition that the acceptable daily intake (ADI) has been followed.[27]

Of course, this also initiated more massive scientific researches on the relationship *aspartame-cancer* but with a different subject of the studies this time – humans.

In the first research of that kind from 2006, conducted by the National Cancer Institute (NCI) scientists, almost *half a million* men and women (between the age of 50 and 71) were studied. They were consuming different types of drinks containing aspartame on a daily basis. The results of that huge work didn't show any development of cancer cells – directly or indirectly related to the intake of the artificial sweetener.[28]

In 2013, probably the most significant work on the topic was published – a detailed meta-analysis of a great number of studies related to the aspartame safety to humans for the period 1990-2012. A team of five of the best international experts was hired to conduct this analysis. And if someone is now skeptical about the true motives of research of such a scale, you don't have to worry – it was sponsored by the Italian Association for Cancer Research. In other words, people who were highly interested in examining that topic.

The conclusion of the team of scientists was more than explicit – aspartame does NOT cause any kind of cancer, digestive problems, diabetes or cardiovascular problems provided that we don't exceed the acceptable daily intake of it.[29]

So, let's put an end to all of the speculations about the relation between cancer and aspartame. Since so far these proved to be only speculations, lies, and myths.

No such relation has ever been found.

Apart from the studies and researches in question, on the Internet, you can easily find dozens of other scientific works and *none* of them has reached conclusions that could shock us.

Aspartame and other "side effects"

However, despite that, a lot of people still don't trust science.

They claim that no matter what scientists say, they simply don't feel well after taking aspartame and that's that!

Some of them complain of headaches (we already discussed that case), others feel some fatigue, yet others are nauseated and so on.

These symptoms made a group of scientists wonder if, by any chance, there are people among us who really cannot *tolerate* that substance.

And that's why, in 2015, they did an interesting test – they gathered two groups of volunteers of about fifty people – the first group claimed they didn't tolerate aspartame much and they had unpleasant symptoms after taking it. The other group shared they didn't have any issues when consuming the artificial sweetener. The scientists told the two groups that they gave them aspartame twice a day and they would record the results. What they didn't share with the groups, however, was that from time to time they gave them a placebo product instead of aspartame.

And indeed – the "sensitive" towards aspartame people immediately reported some unpleasant symptoms after the intake of the sweetener. However, they complained even when they took the placebo product which didn't contain aspartame...[30]

To be completely sure in their conclusions, the scientists took blood and urine samples from those who complained to check if aspartame metabolized correctly.

It turned out at the end that there were no issues at all, aspartame was metabolized perfectly normal with the people in both test groups.

In other words, the reported symptoms were just placebo – people who thought they were aspartame intolerant reacted *psychologically* to the idea that they consumed aspartame, even though they didn't take it at all.

Therefore, if it happens to you to feel some strange symptoms after aspartame consumption, please make sure that these symptoms are *real* and you're not just paranoid about taking the substance. You might need to search for ways to fix your consciousness – actually, this whole chapter might be a good start for that.

Haters gonna hate

I don't know if you've paid attention that only in this chapter we used more than 20 scientific works and conclusions of world organizations and associations which have reported many times the same result – the artificial sweetener aspartame is a substance that is *completely safe* to consume provided we don't have any suicidal thoughts and decide to drink dozens of liters of soft drinks every day.

As a matter of fact, aspartame is one of the most *examined* substances... ever! But how does it happen that it cannot strengthen its position as a safe ingredient among people despite the tons of scientific information that guarantees its safety (when taken reasonably)?

I wonder if the common belief that if something is too good to be true, it's simply not true doesn't play any part. To be honest, the fact itself that there is a substance that is sweeter than sugar and doesn't contain any calories indeed sounds way too good.

But it's true – thanks to the miracles of modern technology and science, we can afford the same sweet taste without any worries about calories or any other health risks.

The hidden risks

Still, the coin always has two sides.

Even though it has been proven that aspartame is safe to humans, consuming it way too often might easily lead to bad eating and behavioral *habits*, especially with people who are already following some diet.

From a behavioral point of view, the aspartame and the diet drinks could encourage people to take more calories in as some people often feel they need to have a Big Mac or a piece of cheesecake as a "moral reward" for drinking only water and zero-calorie drinks all day long. Thus, believing they can afford that treat, they often allow themselves to become more inconsistent with their diets and respectively, to slow or even worsen their results.

Moreover, consuming such zero-calorie drinks with artificial sweeteners too often encourages our brain and taste buds to *seek* the sweet taste simply because our taste preferences are based on our long experience with a given taste.[31]

And while this isn't much of a problem with drinks with no calories, the situation with the sweet foods is quite different.

If a can of diet coke is a precondition for having also a piece of a cake, this must alert us that the "side effect" of the sweetener has been activated. Yes, a small piece of a cake from time to time could be a positive influence from a psychological and social point of view, but unfortunately, a lot of people cannot get satiated only with it and before they even realize it, they're in a situation that destroys their whole dieting plan.

The big picture

And yet – the conclusion is that aspartame is safe, tasty, affordable, and with zero calories.

It has been examined long enough and *way* too many times so that we can trust it and use it as an additional tool when building a healthier lifestyle focused not only on the final physical results and improved health biomarkers but also on mental and social pleasure during the whole process of achieving them.

Superfoods or superhype?

The difference between Superman and the rest of the ordinary men is that he's a superhero with superpowers who always take care of the weak ones or saves those in danger of death. All Metropolis citizens admire him and love him. He's one of a kind and his unique and exceptional power is never doubted. This is all very good but there is one "tiny" problem – Superman is nothing but a very well-made *fiction*.

The comparison between Superman and the other ordinary people could be also applied for the "superfoods" and the other, let's call them, "ordinary" foods.

"Superfoods" are considered to have magical qualities – it's believed that they will cure us of all sorts of illnesses, they will help us win the endless war with kilograms, and they will keep us safe. "Superfoods" are exotic, rare, expensive and precious – not everyone has the privilege to include them regularly in their meals. "Superfoods" are thought to be the greatest food wealth and the mystical ingredient for strong health.

But are they, just like Superman, a perfectly made-up fiction or not?

For that purpose, we'll need to go further back in time – back to the dawn of the industrial age.

At that point, human labor was gradually replaced by machines and manufacturing started to automate. The regionally grown crops started to spread all over the world and the crops reached unprecedented levels. Thus, over time, people had more and more access to products and services, and on top of that, these were even more affordable. In this way, people satisfied their need to consume more and more often.

At a certain point, however, the food industry realized that a new approach was needed for the sales to continue. And in the meantime, people started to pay more and more attention to their looks and health – and it was something that the producers and market analysts welcomed with open arms.

More or less, this was the main reason for the food products to begin to *diversify* – new, never seen before products appeared – gluten-free, low-fat, zero-calorie, organic products. So, the ordinary, conventional ones even started to be considered not that healthy because of that strong diversification. The common belief that if a person wants to be healthy, they'll have to pay a higher price for the very same healthy products, was getting stronger. Logically, this means that the ones who produced and sold those healthy products would have higher profits, as well.

But is this also the case with the superfoods? Are they the next pseudo-healthy food category that aims at satisfying our latest whim or there is truly something very valuable, healthy and special in those foods?

The first superfood?

After quickly going through the industrial revolution period and understanding the reasons behind product diversification, we gradually reached the period of World War I.

The American United Fruit Company became extremely popular at that time and it was one of the biggest food industry monopolies in the USA. The key point here is that during that period, the company controlled around 50% of the *banana* trade and was the prime importer of the fruit in the States.

And when dealing with such a serious business, flawless advertising, without a doubt, should have been on point as well.

Therefore, the marketers that worked for the United Fruit Company, started a massive advertising campaign that aimed at familiarizing the American citizens with the nutritional wealth of bananas. Some very good-looking and highly professional brochures were created which told in great details the precious characteristics of bananas – how practical for every diet they were, how full of nutrients they were, how easy to digest they were, how affordable they were and how easy to consume raw or cooked they were. Special attention was paid even to their peel and the fact that it was the banana's natural "shield".

The brochure they named "Banana Nutritional Values" became tremendously popular.[32]

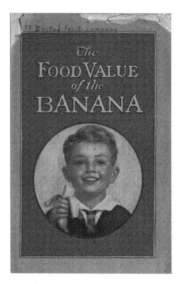

The power of marketing
Source: library.nyam.org

Its content encouraged people to consume the healthy fruit at any time of the day and to include it in all their meals.

Unsurprisingly, these ads brought a lot of success. The banana craze was started, and it even continued in the years after these campaigns when some scientists who got deeply interested in the fruit, found a relation between the intake of bananas and the reduced risk of celiac disease and diabetes (a brief note here – back then, people were still *not* familiar with gluten).

So, people literally went mad with these "discoveries" – of course, all kinds of banana diets started back then and the price of the fruit went up immediately. But this didn't stop the sales from going up, as well. And this was simply because ads did their job.

And even though the actual term *"superfood"* had not been directly used in the advertising materials, the idea for such a product had already been born – a type of food that cures, that is new, luxurious and tasty. Simply said – better than all the rest.

However, as if nowadays the glory of banana has been waning. Even though they're amongst the fruits with the highest levels of potassium[33], the high calories they provide scare away a lot of the people who follow a certain diet. Mostly, the people who follow the extremely famous keto diet.

What's trendy today?

It's interesting to observe the trend of superfoods – it could be easily classified as *cyclic* because, in different periods, different types of superfoods have been favorized.

The situation is identical to the one in clothes and fashion, don't you think?

For example, a few years ago, (2013-2016)[34], *goji berry* was the most popular (and respectively – "healthiest") fruit – it was in high demand, bought, consumed and recommended by all sorts of celebrities and nutritionists. Its characteristics were widely discussed and confirmed in a lot of magazines and websites for healthy eating and living.

However, sometime around 2017, people started talking less and less about the fruit, it wasn't always included in every diet, and its healthy super-characteristics were somehow forgotten.

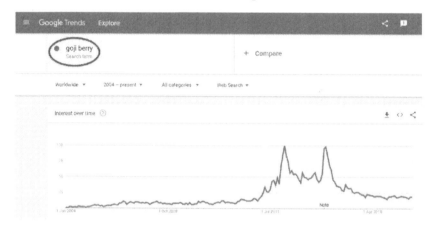

Peaked all of a sudden; died all of a sudden
Source: Google Trends

Of course, this doesn't mean that ten years from now the goji berries wouldn't get trendy again.

But speaking about what's trendy today, it'd make sense to evaluate in more detail some of the "superfoods" of our time, right?

I suspect that everyone would agree that they've seen information about how genuinely healthy *blueberries, avocado,* and *quinoa* are. They're all presented if not as mandatory, at least as highly recommended food products that should be included regularly in our menu.

As foods with significantly better nutritional values than all other foods; as foods that will protect us from sickness and help us stay in a good shape; as "superfoods".

Blueberry

Let's begin with *blueberries* – apart from being so tasty, affordable and with low calories, they're best known for being a great source of *antioxidants.*

And we've all heard how antioxidants help eliminate the free radicals in our bodies and that's why they're believed to be super healthy. For many years the US Department of Agriculture (USDA) stated that blueberries are top food ("superfood") when it comes to quantity of antioxidants.

Nowadays, however, it's well-known that free radicals are, in fact, one of the immune system weapons when coping with all kinds of pathogens and even some cancers. For that reason, having them *completely* neutralized in our bodies isn't something that we need to strive to achieve by all means.

Talking about antioxidants, scientists found a few other interesting things.

First, it turned out that they have a large number of other properties related to fighting free radicals, beyond the ones that have been known – these are properties that are still to be analyzed and examined further though.[35]

In other words, there are many other questions about antioxidants that are still waiting for a clear answer.

Second, science has proven that *anthocyanins* and *flavonoids* (which are the antioxidants in blueberries), in fact, have almost *no* antioxidant qualities. These substances get metabolized in our bodies so fast that their healthy antioxidant properties, in practice, don't have the necessary time to be expressed.[36]

Of course, this isn't valid when we talk about an *in vitro* environment, where their qualities are much stronger, but, in the end, it's important what's happening *in vivo* (in our organism), isn't it?

I'd like to quickly clarify something important – I hope you don't have any dark thoughts regarding blueberries as food – they're indeed a great, great fruit – low in calories, tasty and rich in micronutrients.

However, can we consider them to be better when compared with raspberries or blackberries, for instance?

And this is exactly where the exaggeration starts.

Take raspberries and blackberries - they're both a cut above blueberries in a few significant aspects - they're *less* in calories, they have *more* dietary fibers, *more* vitamin C and *more* manganese.[37] [38] [39]

Parameter (per 100 g)	Blueberry	Raspberry	Blackberry
Calories	57	**52**	62
Dietary fibers (g)	2.4	6.5	**7.6**
Vitamin C (mg)	9.7	26.2	**30.2**
Vitamin K (mcg)	19.3	7.8	**28.5**
Manganese (mg)	0.3	0.7	**0.9**

Still, the "superfood" winner is... blueberry

But, most probably, you don't hear often raspberries and blackberries being classified as "superfoods".

Avocado

Unnoticeably, we've reached the second product of the short "super list" – a very well-known green fruit which has surely not become popular overnight – *avocado*.

Apart from the specific nutritional qualities that will be discussed right in the next paragraph, this fruit is very practical too – we can easily include it in all kinds of soups, juices, toasts, salads, smoothies. Indeed, few are the food products that could be consumed in so many ways.

However, what truly distinguishes avocado from the other fruits is the number of *fats* it has. A single avocado contains nearly 30 grams of fat, 20 grams of which are *monounsaturated* fats.

In other words, the kind of fats that we need to consume the most as they've been proven to have many health benefits.

Nevertheless, the monounsaturated fats aren't the only good surprise that avocado offers – it's also a great source of dozens of other microelements – vitamins C, E, and K, potassium, and others.

We shouldn't also underestimate the fact that one avocado has 13 grams of *fiber* – and that certainly makes for an impressive micronutrient profile![40]

Unfortunately, there is always a "*but*"! Because no matter how tasty, widely used and rich in nutrients avocado is, it does have *high* calories.

Really high calories.

A single avocado contains about 300 calories – indeed, all of them are coming from healthy sources, but calories are calories after all, and this is an energy that our body takes in no matter what.

Just as a comparison – two large bananas have significantly lower calories than a single medium in size avocado.

1 avocado (~200 g)	2 large bananas (270 g)
322 kcal	242 kcal

Now probably some will have a reason to express their indignation – *"Yet, a lot of people don't eat a whole avocado per day, they only eat half of it, for example!"*

That's true, but if we look at the things from that perspective – yes, half an avocado means half the calories, but it also means half the Omega 3 and 6 fatty acids, half the vitamins, half the minerals, half the fibers. Correct?

Apart from that, many of us like making fancy-looking and sophisticated meals, where part of the recipe is just that small half of an avocado. The seed often gets removed and is then filled with various creative appetizers, cheese, sauces, etc.

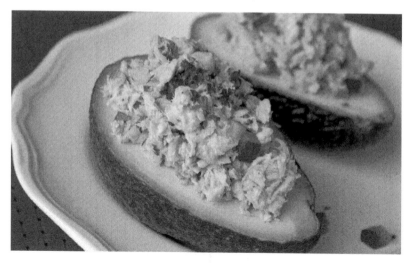

Healthy? Yes! Tasty? Yes! Calorie-dense? YES!
Source: traderjoes.com

And suddenly, the two super tasty and super healthy bites of that stuffed avocado turn out to be a meal that not only isn't voluminous and satiating but also containing 300+ calories at the same time.

Another rarely mentioned disadvantage is that avocado is among the fruits that aren't *appropriate* to be consumed by everyone.

Almost half of the people who have a *latex allergy*, for instance, also have highly distinguished *intolerance* to that fruit[41] which leads to symptoms such as eyes and lips bloating, lips or throat itching, sneezing and all different types of skin and stomach problems.

According to data published a few years ago by Harvard Health Publishing, around 60% of the world population has high intolerance or is allergic to latex.[42] In other words, people who have to be on their guard when consuming avocado appear to be a significant number.

I hope you understand me correctly – avocado is an exceptional fruit and you can eat it every day and this by no means would be a wrong decision. Especially if you take into consideration the amounts that you consume.

Is it right to define it as a "superfood" though?

A far better definition would be a "high-calorie superfood".

However, this doesn't sound that sexy, does it?

Quinoa

We have now reached the last (but of course not least) important "superfood" from our brief list – *quinoa*.

This grain crop (let's not confuse it with a wheat crop) surprisingly or not, gained its popularity during the years when *gluten* had made a stir. This is no accident in fact, as quinoa doesn't contain any gluten in contrast to almost all other foods that contain starch. Or at least the quantity of gluten in quinoa doesn't cause any issues to those that are somewhat intolerant to it. Because of that, it's considered safe for most of us who are gluten sensitive or have been diagnosed with celiac disease.

So, we admit a point for quinoa here - Super-quinoa vs. Super-fiction – 1:0.

Quinoa is known to be a "superfood" because of its rich nutrient and protein profile too.

In other words, the protein in quinoa contains *all* the essential amino acids. Such protein profile is found only in animal products and quinoa is just one of the very few exceptions from the large family of plants.

Besides, it's a very good source of magnesium, phosphorus, and manganese.[43]

Therefore, let's give another point for quinoa – Super-quinoa vs. Super-fiction – 2:0.

Regardless of its complete protein profile, quinoa doesn't contain a lot of protein in general.

100 grams of boiled quinoa has a little bit more than 4 grams of protein which could certainly be determined as low quantity, especially for those who actively do sports.

The rest of the macronutrients are mainly carbs - and fibers, which in 100 grams of the product don't even reach 3 grams.

Just for comparison, 100 grams of boiled beans have an almost identical number of calories, but the quantities of protein and fibers are *double*.[44]

Parameter (per 100 g)	Boiled quinoa	Boiled beans
Calories (kcal)	120	127
Protein (g)	4.4	**8.7**
Dietary fibers (g)	2.8	**6.4**
Magnesium (mg)	**64**	42
Phosphorus (mg)	**152**	138

Still, quinoa is on a pedestal

So, it'd be fair to give a point to the other "team" here – Super-quinoa vs. Super-fiction – 2:1.

Despite its notable micronutrient profile, quinoa manages to "keep" all of its healthy agents to itself. It's a well-known fact that the quantity of nutrients from a given food that is absorbed by human bodies *isn't* the same quantity of nutrients that the food has. To a great extent, this is due to the number of *antinutrients* that many foods have.

In the case with quinoa, these are the so-called *phytates* – they're a type of an antinutrient that interfere with the absorption of certain minerals. They block the total absorption mainly of the minerals zinc, iron, phosphorus, and magnesium – that's almost all the microelements found in high quantities in quinoa.

And this is a great disadvantage here – the quantity of that antinutrient in quinoa is very high.[45] [46] And even though we can cope with that problem to some extent by soaking the raw quinoa in warm water with lemon juice or apple vinegar for a few hours to reduce its the phytic acid content[47], yet we cannot get rid of the antinutrients *completely*.

So, it turns out that the high micronutrient profile of quinoa is only on paper. And for that, we should give a new point to Super-fiction which makes the current result of the "battle" draw – Super-quinoa vs. Super-fiction – 2:2.

But this is not the end at all.

Similar to many other "superfoods", the popularity of quinoa caused a rise in its price, too.

In the trustworthy website *Tridge.com*, you can easily check the average global stock price of almost any food product, including quinoa.

On 24th July 2019, the global price of a kilo of quinoa was $2.32 (with a tendency to go up).[48]

As a contrast, the price of white rice was only $0.71[49], of corn - $0.50[50] and of millet - $0.27.[51]

These are all foods that could be consumed instead of quinoa, but yet they aren't classified as "superfoods".

And even if we do accept that in some aspects quinoa is healthier than the foods mentioned, we cannot firmly state that it's more than 5 times better than them. The price of quinoa, however, is 5 times higher than the one of the other foods.

$uperfoods & #superfoods

As we see, neither blueberries are many times better than raspberries and blackberries, nor is quinoa much healthier than white rice or beans. Avocado, on the other side, is unique in many ways but we might take into consideration the high calories it has and not go to extremes with it. Things that seem far from the expected characteristics of something that is presented as super healthy, right?

Truth is simple, but yet hard to accept by the majority – "superfood" is simply an advertising *label* and marketing *tool*.

There is no clear *officially acclaimed* scientific definition for the products in question. *No one* in the scientific fields – neither scientists nor nutritionists, use that term.

It comes to that Regulation 1924/2006 of the European Union. It sought to regulate the claims on foods labeled and advertised in the EU as it practically *banned* the advertising of products labeled as "superfoods" if they aren't supported by scientifically-based evidence that guaranteed the claimed health benefits and characteristics.[52]

The result of that decision is not surprising at all – today, you can hardly see a label on a food product (at least, I haven't seen such in Europe) that presents the given product as a "superfood".

And if the manufacturers had the opportunity to advertise their goods as "superfood", then they'd surely do that, no doubt about that. Yet, this cannot happen as the law requires direct evidence – and that is simply... missing.

Nevertheless, people still seem to be uninterested in that – they always want to find that universal food which will satiate all their nutritional needs. It doesn't matter to them that a truly healthy diet, in its complete essence, should contain plenty of *different* sources of nutrients.

Indeed, the so-called "superfoods" also have their major place in a good, healthy diet but placing them on a pedestal isn't justified.

But favoring them has reached such heights that consuming "superfoods" is nowadays considered a *social* rather than health need. There is nothing cooler than preparing the sophisticated and exotic salad of the TV show celebrity, taking a photo of it and posting it on Instagram - the *#superfood* hashtag is mandatory.

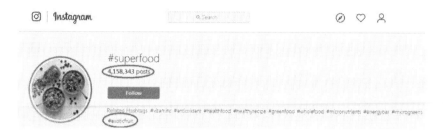

Over 4 million #superfood posts in Instagram. Related hashtag: #exoticfruit
It's not a coincidence.

Yet, a photo of a meal of beans and spearmint cannot get enough likes on social media.

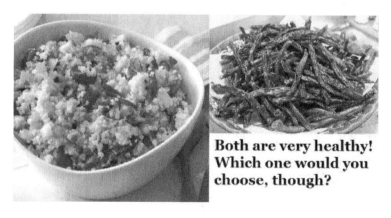

Both are very healthy!
Which one would you
choose, though?

We've now reached the point when consuming exotic, organic and "superfoods" demonstrates a high social *status* and is part of the list with un-written rules on how to be part of modern society.

Don't you already notice that?

All the famous "influencers" eat only gluten-free, organic foods, the ones that are trendy now, *at this very moment.*

65

At the same time, "ordinary" people gobble with corn with mayonnaise and offal.

That way of thinking is simply wrong and restrictive.

A hidden gem

Mentioning offal, I'd like to talk about one particular food that contains so many vitamins and minerals in an amazing proportion of macronutrients as no other "trendy" "superfood" at the moment.

It might sound odd, but I'm talking about *chicken livers*.

They turn out to be a real micronutrient "bomb" – they have a high content of vitamins A, C, B1, B2, B3, B5, B6, B9, and B12; iron, phosphorus, selenium, zinc, copper, manganese, choline.[53]

They have an incredible and complete amino-acid profile.

And they're rich in proteins.

They're low in calories.

They satiate us.

They're easy to cook.

They're tasty.

Then, why don't chicken livers have that status of stardom as all of the foods that we've discussed so far?

And it's not about them only – beef and pork livers are also quite similar as characteristics but, sadly, as popularity too.

But let's be honest – livers, in general, aren't very... *sexy* food, are they? They're simply not the type of product that could sell nowadays. They're cheap and affordable. They aren't good-looking. They aren't wrapped up in some mysticism and they don't have millennial history.

They aren't rare. They're ordinary. They're boring. And let's not forget the fact that they're an animal product, so they're not the food of choice for all the vegans and vegetarians around the world.

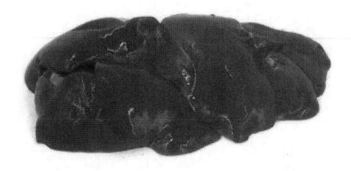

This will never be a "superfood"... look at it – it's UGLY!

Many people reading the above will start rumbling: *"What are you talking about, livers are cholesterol bombshell ready to explode!"* or *"They contain toxins, what kind of a crazy idea is that?"*

Cholesterol and toxins do need separate chapters, but, fortunately, they have both been already discussed in the first book of the *"Enjoy Food"* series.

The big picture

Nowadays, people are constantly being convinced that they lack all different kinds of nutrients and the solution to get them is to consume many different "superfoods".

We're somehow often shown in different ways that the successful, rich, healthy person eats only that type of foods – prestigious, outstanding, the ones showing high class and good, sophisticated taste.

While the poor, unsuccessful and ill people eat the "boring", "ordinary" foods.

And before we realize it, we're already faced with a major *"food discrimination"* that confuses the ones who simply want to start living more healthily and maybe lose some weight. That "food discrimination" makes it hard for them to tell which product is a true "superfood" and which isn't.

It was only yesterday when goji berries were considered "superfood", too, and now that privilege is granted to acai berries, for instance.

Some sources state that a certain food X is "superfood" and other sources claim the opposite – that it's "super evil".

Where is the truth?

At the same time, people with financial difficulties are getting demotivated as they believe they cannot live healthily because they cannot afford the "superfoods".

So, instead of focusing on "superfoods", it'd be much more reasonable to think about the best possible *"supermeal"* that you can afford.

A meal that is *balanced* in calories, fibers, proteins, fats, vitamins, minerals, and taste. This is what our body wants and what would be beneficial for it over time.

Indeed, that "supermeal" could include blueberries or quinoa but it'd be efficient enough if it also has rice or blackberries.

Yes, that "supermeal" might cost you $15, but it might be $5, too.

But regardless of the differences, the resemblance is always the same – *every* food in a true "supermeal" could be our "superfood".

WhATER?

Speaking about healthy habits, nourishing food, and sport, we can surely spare some time on the most essential element of life – *water*.

When it comes to significance, it explicitly beats any type of food. And that was well-known even back in the ancient days – people back then even worshipped it because of their beliefs, mythology, and folklore. And even though it has always been depicted as a source of life, they never forgot that it might also be a force of destruction.

Despite the great influence water had on their minds in that period of the development of human civilization, people were not able to explain to themselves what makes water so essential.

The very first records of its study are found in ancient Greece. The philosopher Thales of Miletus recognized water as one of the four main elements of nature that made up all matter (along with earth, fire, and air). That point of view was also supported by Plato two centuries later.

It got a lot more exciting in the 18th century when the English scientist Henry Cavendish found a substance which, when reacting with oxygen created... pure water. It was then clear that water isn't just an "element" of nature but an actual chemical compound.

Some years later, the French chemist Antoine Lavoisier reproduced Cavendish's work and then gave a name to that compound – *hydrogen* (from the Greek for "water-former").[54]

And so, we move forward to the present days when science has now discovered all the fundamental reasons for the key role of water for the existence of all organisms.

We already know that it's a very strong dissolving agent – all organic compounds are dissolved equally well in it – fats, carbohydrates, proteins, acids, bases, salts, and even some gases.

On top of that, water is hardly ever involved in any undesired chemical reactions with the substances dissolved in it.

We also know a lot more about its thermal conductivity, about the polarity of its molecule, and many other characteristics.

The rapid development of modern technologies, social networks, and the endless, easy-to-access, and free (dis/mis)information, however, made us aware of some new "facts" about water.

In this chapter, we'll dig deeper into them and see what the scientific approach is - and what should be our actions towards them.

How much to drink?

Without a doubt, the topic that has always been discussed the most is how much water *exactly* we need to drink each day to stay healthy.

The belief that we need (at least) 8 glasses per day is perhaps, the most widely spread.

A consumption, based on gender is also circulating out there – for example, 2 liters for men and 1.5 liters for women. Some people declare a person's physical activity as a variable in the equation too.

And from that point on, the mess starts getting serious as all sorts of discussions, calculations and brain teasers are initiated.

We're getting provided with different physical activity scales and then different scales of the *intensity* of that activity. Over time, more and more criteria are taken into account - age, body type, weight, stress levels, sweating intensity and even our overall mood.

And our only job is to manually enter all these personal parameters in this complex "calculator" so that we could finally see the holy number of optimal liters of water that we need to drink.

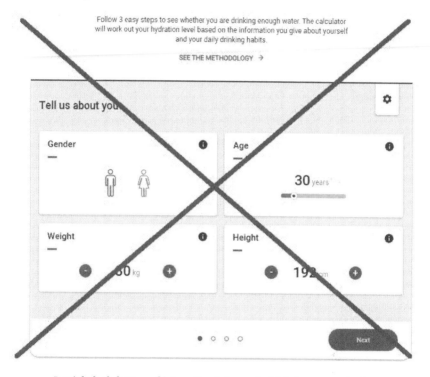

It might look fancy and interesting to know, but it brings no real value

But what happens if we start losing weight (or gaining weight)?

And what happens just a year later, when we get older?

Well, come on, it shouldn't be a problem at all – we'll just re-calculate everything yet again...

Besides, nowadays we can even find numerous mobile apps that would kindly remind us to drink our water. It's easy - we simply set the interval of time that we want the phone to remind us to hydrate. And after we drink the glass of water, of course, we click on the fancy button to mark this done.

And if by any chance, we're at a place where we don't have a supply of water when the phone sends its reminder, we try to remember that alert and when we finally have the chance to drink some water, we drink double the amount. You know, because we need to compensate...

No matter what we say, this could be *huge* mental torture happening on a daily basis - constantly thinking about the lack of hydration, counting the number of glasses, and eventually feeling unwell if things just don't go as planned.

The good news is that it isn't really necessary. At all.

Truth is that, so far, not a *single* scientifically-proven reason to drink a certain minimum amount of water has been found.

That has been documented ever since the beginning of the 2000s just to be verified many times in the years after.[55] [56] [57]

In 2005, the Medicine institute of the American National Academy of Science stated that *"while it might appear useful to estimate an average requirement (an EAR) for water, an EAR based on data is not possible."*[58]

But even if we *hypothetically* agree that we could somehow understand the exact amount of our daily water needs, our actual intake would *still* be compromised. Because we consume water through all the different kinds of beverages and even the food that we eat.

Yes, everything that we *eat*, contains some water. Especially, when we eat foods that are rich in nutrients – mainly, fruit and vegetables.

A quite interesting scientific publication from 2004 stated that around 20% of the water that we take during the day, in fact, comes from our food.[59]

Food	Amount of water in 100 g (g)
Orange	86.7
Kale	84.5
Chicken breast, raw	74.8
Quinoa, uncooked	13.3
Avocado	73.2
White bread, commercially prepared	30.4
White mushrooms, raw	92.4

Source: nutritiondata.com

Therefore, instead of constantly thinking about how much to drink, waiting for some reminders from your phone and feeling distressed whenever you don't have some water around you, just trust your best integrated "alarm" – your *thirst*.

It's simple – whenever you feel slightly thirsty, just drink water.

And if you're at a place where you don't have access to water and you feel that thirst for a bit longer, it's okay, don't panic. Because when you finally get some water, the accumulated thirst will automatically force your body to drink more to compensate.

There is no point in becoming a maniac and losing your nerves over some "magic" consumption formula that simply doesn't work in the way we think it does.

And let's not ignore that drinking water is also related to feeling *pleasure*. And satisfying your thirst is, surely, one of the greatest pleasures, don't you agree?

Lemon water

And yet, it's true that millions of people are now starting to forget the joy of drinking the regular tap water.

They get inspired by some external stimuli and decide to do some good to their bodies by adding something "fresh" to their water – most often lime or lemon.

In recent years, the consumption of *lemon water* transformed from a standard taste preference into a real health-related hype.[60] That, of course, happened not without the help of some popular celebrity doctors and other well-known (and not that well-known) people.

It feels right to say here that I mind neither lemons nor water, not lemon water. Lemons are wonderful fruit, drinking water is great, and lemon water has a very nice taste – it's all true.

I'm just skeptical about all the recognition and hype that lemon water is getting. It's not some *miracle* water, and there is nothing *special* about it. It's nothing better than the "boring", "old-fashioned" tap water that we could drink.

And fortunately, science also supports that statement.

There is no better start than the one related to the most popular belief - lemon water helps about *weight loss*.

It's surely not a coincidence that the majority of the supporters of this belief are those who also support all the detox regimes (we'll discuss this in a bit). According to the supporters of this statement, stopping any kind of food for a certain short period along with a high intake of lemon water results in a quick, noticeable, and healthy weight loss.

I've been talking with lots of people who swear in the correctness of that statement.

But it's more than ridiculous.

Just to mention it yet again - the *only* condition for losing weight is to consume *less energy* than the energy that our body spends.

Let's use a simple logic here - what happens when we stop eating food and only drink water (either with limes, lemons or cucumbers)? Well, what happens is that we simply stop taking *any* energy. In other words – we put ourselves in, literally, the most aggressive (and far from healthy) caloric deficit.

And yes, therefore our body will start to lose weight quite rapidly. But what we'll lose as weight would NOT be body fat - it'd be mainly water and muscle mass. Besides, our glycogen stores will get completely emptied.[61] And when we return to normal eating (because we should start eating again someday), water would also come back, the glycogen stores would quickly get filled and the scale would show (in the best case scenario) the same weight that we so hard aimed to reduce.

Still, some don't go on detox diets but yet they drink lemon water for the sole purpose of losing weight more easily. They argue that the higher intake of water before meals make them eat less. And the pleasant lemon taste just helps them drinking more water.

To be honest, even though there is some sense in that thesis, science has confirmed in many studies that the same effect (to eat less) could also be achieved by drinking regular water.[62 63 64 65]

Simply said, it's nothing more than a simple taste *preference* – it's been proven that the "seasoned" water has no additional benefits when compared with the regular water when it comes to losing weight.

Another popular belief about lemon water is that it supports body *detoxification*. Even if we don't go into details about the completely wrong perception about human physiology that is represented by the so-called "detox" (completely unraveled in the first book of the *"Enjoy Food"* series), this statement still makes no logic.

Maybe the nutrients or some other bioactive agents that lemon has, could affect the detoxifying enzymes of our liver?

Maybe.

Unfortunately, at the moment these are only *speculations* and there is *no* direct evidence to support the suggestion.

The only records that we have are just a few studies that were conducted a few decades ago on *lab mice in an in vitro environment* where a similar effect was indeed reported with the *limonene* molecule (yes, quite an attractive name).[66] But the degree to which the attainable dozes of limonene or other lemon ingredients could stimulate the liver to better detoxify the human body, is still unknown. In other words, even if we *hypothetically* agree that lemons could support the work of the liver, this would be observed (again, eventually) if the intake of the fruit is *extremely* high.

So, in practice, this enormous "advantage" of lemon water remains... a myth.

There is also no possible way not to talk more about the common misconception that the lemon water is a great support in the fight against malignant formations.

Those who promote that idea, at first sight, seem to provide some reasonable explanation but just a bit of common sense and verification of the facts is needed to have all this easily disproven.

All in all, it's believed that an *acidic* environment in our body could significantly *increase* the chance of cancer cells to develop. For this acidic environment to happen, the blood pH must drop under the normal levels of 7.35-7.45 units.

And the idea of the lemon water proponents (and the proponents of the *alkaline diet*, in general) is for this drop to never happen – that is to say, to maintain higher pH levels of the blood with the help of "alkaline" foods and "alkaline" water.

But this is a game more threatening than playing with fire – it's medically proven that even the slightest changes out of the normal levels of the blood pH could have irreversible and even fatal consequences to our organism. For instance, if your blood pH increases to 7.8 and above or goes down to 6.8 and below, this would be... lethal for you.[67]

Blood pH Levels

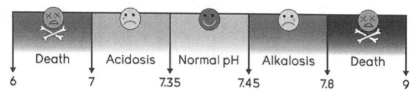

| Death | Acidosis | Normal pH | Alkalosis | Death |

6   7   7.35   7.45   7.8   9

Source: cairopedneph.com

The inexplicable thing is the common conception that water with lemons has "alkaline" qualities. Even though lemon juice produces minimal quantities of alkaline metabolites, it consists only of *citrate* (lemon acid) that has low pH – 2 or 3 units.

And there is *no* possible way for *acid* to *alkalize* anything.

The whole idea just crashes into pieces here.

Anyhow, we've already touched upon the *alkaline diets* – I'd like to briefly say something here. The practitioners of that type of eating must take into consideration that our body aims to always stay in a stable, relatively constant internal environment, called *homeostasis*.

And that homeostasis couldn't be changed by the outer environment. Simply said, our body maintains unchanged its inner environment so that it guarantees the smooth and effective course of all the biological processes that go in it.

The pH of the inner environment (that is to say, blood) CANNOT be changed by eating or drinking any type of food. And that is maintained and regulated by all the buffer systems that keep the acid levels in our bodies steady and don't allow any outside factors to influence the homeostasis.[68] [69]

And no, this does NOT slow down our bodies in any way.

Our bodies aren't hampered by the meat or eggs that we eat, or any other "acidic" food, but by the whole *unhealthy lifestyle* that we live.

And when people who have eaten so far only burgers, chips and pizza, suddenly start following the alkaline diet and simply feel the positive sides of consuming less processed foods, this pleasant feeling isn't related to any imaginary change of the blood pH but is related with the overall positive change in their eating habits.

And yet – as with all the other diets, at least we have some indirect positive effect in the end – despite the wrong motives, people are *still* stimulated to consume more fruits and vegetables. On the other hand, however, a lot of healthy products, most of them – rich in proteins, are unfairly demonized.

So, let's put an end to the whole debate about the water with a taste. You'll neither lose weight more easily by drinking it nor will you improve your health in any way or protect yourself from any insidious disease.

And yet, this book is all about enjoying food, and diets... and drinks. Therefore, if you really like the taste of water with lemon/lime/cucumber/whatever - then, go ahead, drink it like this.

You prefer the usual tap water? Again – there is no problem at all.

Raw water

Talking about the tap water and the one with a taste, unfortunately, there are still many more different "types" of water out there.

A great part of them is proclaimed as extremely healthy, even sometimes *miraculous*. Over some other types, however, a dark shadow has been cast – the interesting part is that the most traduced one is the standard tap water. Not that it's harmful or something else, but according to some people, it simply doesn't provide all the extras that "modern" waters have.

And one of these "newly-found" ones is the so-called *raw* water.

It reached the peak of its popularity at the beginning of 2018, however, all the advantages of that type of hydrogen oxide were almost immediately disproved and its glorious life was put to an end shortly afterward.[70]

Despite that, even to this date, there is still a lot of support for the consumption of raw water. But in contrast to the lemon water, here things aren't just a matter of taste preferences - they could be very *dangerous*.

So, what's raw water? Its consumers eagerly explain that one of the ways to stay optimally healthy is to consume mainly *natural* products that haven't undergone *any* technology treatments.

They believe that raw water is as close as possible to the water found in wild nature, which, as they share, is the purest and least contaminated, and at the same time, contained healthy bacteria and minerals. Because of those reasons, some people prefer to turn their backs to the tap water and turn to the water from natural water basins.

Four words here – *do not do this*!

The beliefs of those people couldn't be more *wrong*. Not only water in nature isn't any better than the one we drink at home, but it might also be a big *threat* for our lives – unfortunately, due to the direct consumption of contaminated water, every year almost half a million people around the world die.[71]

And yes – raw water is far more *contaminated* than the one running in our homes. In the water basins in nature, we can find many forms of life and they're a source of bacterial, fungal and viral contamination - *Escherichia coli, Salmonella spp.* and many others. Their presence in the otherwise „pure" raw water simply indicates that the water in question is, more or less, contaminated with... *feces*.

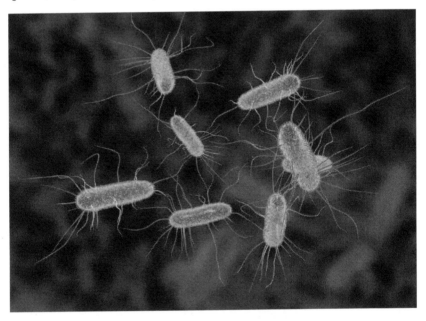

You don't see it... but it's there.
Source: independent.co.uk

Therefore, water should always go through the required quality control so that corrective actions and measures are taken in case of a need. There is no better guarantee for community safety and keeping people healthy than that.

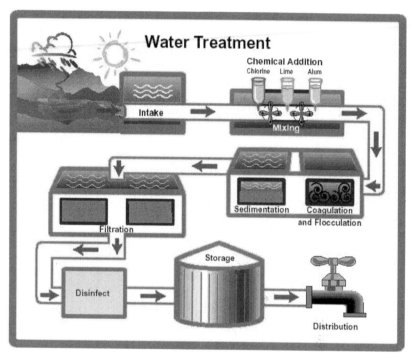

Source: jzcacayuran.wordpress.com

In general, in most of the USA and Europe, the quality of water is under very strict monitoring and we should have no worries about drinking it.

Yet, if you have any doubts regarding the quality of the tap water in your region, you may contact your local water provider and ask them for a verified report outlining the levels of any contamination.

Cold or warm?

Myths and fads concerning water don't stop here - they're way more than you can think of.

And there are those related to its *temperature*.

Those who are about to start their "journey" with popular diets are often advised to drink *warm* water to tame their hunger or appetite.

I don't know about you, but the sole idea of drinking warm water doesn't sound, mildly said, very tempting to me.

Good thing, at least, is that there is *no* scientific paper that has *ever* found *any* relation between hunger/appetite and warm water.

If we'd drink a liter of warm water or a liter of a bit colder water, there would be no difference except in the fact that satisfying our thirst with the warm one would surely be less pleasant.

And this isn't something that should be underestimated.

Here I'd like to give a piece of advice to you to try something which has proven to bring more success. Instead of drinking warm water, just try with *sparkling* water. It'll fill up your stomach and you'll be able to tame your hunger a little bit easier. And it'll also tame the desire for drinking fizzy drinks. In practice, you kill two birds with one stone.

And what people have been saying about *cold* water?

Millions around the globe do consider that the colder the water we drink, the more calories we'd burn, and, respectively, more weight would be lost.

Technically, there is *some* logic behind that.

If we drink cold water, our body will need more energy to warm it up till it reached normal body temperature, therefore – indeed, calories are burnt.

The question is – *how many?*

And the answer to that question is... well, few.

An *insignificant* number.

In the chemistry and biology classes that we had at school, we were taught that our body needs around 37 calories to increase the temperature of 1 ml of water from 0° (right on the freezing point) to 37° C (body temperature).

Nevertheless, we have to make a clear clarification here – the energy that comes from our food is in the form of *kilocalories*. This means that in reality, we need 0.037 of the calorie to increase the temperature of 1 ml of water. And to put it simply, this would mean that if we drink 27 ml of ice-cold water, we'd burn the amazing... 1 calorie.

And what happens if we want to burn the calories of, let's say, two standard candies (~130 cal.)?

Well, we'd need to somehow drink around 3.5 liters of ice-cold water. These are only examples proving that we'd rather die of water *intoxication* (already discussed in more detail in the first book of the series) than losing any weight if we follow the recommendations of such beliefs.

And yet, speaking about losing weight, water is, logically, the best choice for a drink. It's easy to obtain and has no calories. Drinking water could also lead to conditions that would indirectly help in losing weight.

No matter if we drink it ice-cold, just a bit colder or warm.

For example, if we grow the habit of drinking a little bit more water before eating, our stomach would be fuller and we'd tend to eat less food later.

Drinking water during meals

We just mentioned drinking water before or during eating and the truth is that some debates have managed to inculcate in *that* direction as well.

Many people still think that drinking water (or other beverages) during a meal influences our *digestion* in a bad way.

There are also some accusations associated with toxins being accumulated more easily when we mix food and water. Apart from those, there are other statements that drinking water while having a meal, reduces the time the food spends in our stomach. And that is considered to be unhealthy as it's believed that the less time food spends with stomach acids and digestive enzymes, the worse nutrients assimilation would be.

Luckily, *none* of these accusations have been supported by science.

Moreover, a few scientific works that examine in detail the processes in question, firmly confirm that liquids, despite going through the digestive system much faster than food, don't affect the speed of food digestion at all.[72]

In fact, drinking water while eating could even have a *positive* effect on digestion. Water helps big bites go through the gullet much easier. It also helps food moving smoother through the intestinal system. If that process doesn't happen easily and smoothly, we feel the well-known bloating and discomfort of our stomach, and we're even faced with constipation.

And that's not all – it's good to remind the opponents of the whole "drink water with meals" idea, that even while digesting the food, our stomach produces not only gastric juices, electrolytes, digestive enzymes, etc., but also *water*.[73] And *that* water is necessary for the normal functioning of the enzymes in question.

Unfortunately, not that many people even think about the additional benefits of drinking water while eating.

For instance, delaying the next bite of our food for a gulp of water gives our body some extra time to work with the satiety signals and *reduce* the hunger we feel.

Thus, we can avoid unnecessary overeating which, without a doubt, is one of the main reasons for obesity.

That's been demonstrated many times – for example, in a 12-week study, half of the participants were given 0.5 liters of water before or during a meal. For those 12 weeks, they lost more than two kilos, compared to the other part of the participants who didn't manage to do that.[74]

Of course, we should never forget about the exceptions.

For a great part of our kind, drinking water or any other beverages while eating, wouldn't cause any issues with normal digestion.

But for those who suffer from *gastroesophageal reflux disease* (GERD), drinking water while eating food might be a pretty bad idea. This is so as even the smallest amount of liquids might cause some serious pressure in the stomach – one that could usually be caused by a large meal, for example. Even worse, this is a precondition for heartburn which people often neglect, but actually, chronic heartburn might lead to some serious complications.

Water before sleep

The last topic about water consumption that's worth addressing, is the one about whether it's healthy or not to drink 1-2 glasses of water *before sleep*.

The proclaimed benefits are the already well-known body detoxification, digestion optimization, blood circulation improvement while sleeping, etc. Plus that it's an easy way to cope with sweating in the hot summer nights.

And even though drinking water is something that we can do at any time, drinking it right before falling asleep is simply... not the best idea.

Probably you can guess the reason for that, right?

That's right – drinking water before sleep means *interrupting* that sleep to go to the toilet. Which translates into a lot worse *quality* of sleep.

Remember, we're diurnal creatures and our bodies work in a way that we shouldn't feel the need to wake up at night – this guarantees us between 6 and 8 hours of good *continuous* sleep in ideal conditions.

And, believe me, no matter what healthy tricks, protocols or diets you follow, if they're at the expense of the quality of your sleep, you'd simply *never* achieve any positive and long-term results.

It's not only about losing weight at all - sleep deprivation might lead to a lot of health deterioration; a very small part of them are:

- Higher blood pressure
- Increased levels of the "bad" cholesterol
- Gaining weight (just the opposite of what you aim for)
- Increased risk of diabetes
- Increased risk of breast cancer and prostate cancer

- Impaired memory
- Lowered libido
- Increased risk of flu and colds
- Low concentration and increased accidents risk

If you need to start forming healthy habits, you should *always* start with those that not only don't negatively affect your sleep but even *optimize* it.

Definitely, a good start would be to restrict drinking water right before sleep.

Leave that for the day.

The big picture

Satisfying thirst is one of the most pleasant physiological pleasures. But, as with any other kinds of pleasures, there should be some moderation here, too.

Just drink safe, technologically treated water throughout the whole day in the amounts that are enough for you to simply feel well.

If you like, put some lemon, lime, cucumber or anything else at your taste. Drink it freely before eating, while eating, after eating, while doing sports, while walking, warm or cold – everything should depend on your convenience and preferences, and not on the fairy-tales of some "specialist" or anonymous articles on the Internet.

And when you combine all of that with an activity that brings you joy, better sleep and better choice of foods and good social life (related with the consumption of "bad" foods and drinks from time to time), you'd not only start losing the kilos that have bothered you so much but also you'd not even notice how that had happened.

Could science be wrong?

In the entire *"Enjoy Food"* series, we were talking about how we shouldn't trust too readily what we hear on television or read on social media. The information that is found there is often there simply because of financial reasons or reasons related to benefits given to a certain "influencer" or shared between a few people.

That's why we reviewed and relied on many scientific works, shared by reliable and verified journals. We based our recommendations, pieces of advice and ideas on them, we even developed some hypothesis and debunked a good number of nutritional myths. It was all about evidence, researches, analysis, and logic. It had to be science or nothing...

However, *even with* science, there are still some elements that we need to be aware of and pay attention to.

It'd be beneficial, for example, if we knew how to more easily distinguish what type of study had been held and which design was developed better. It'd be good to know how to understand the bigger picture of a certain scientific work and the reasons behind it. And, at the same time, it's important to constantly remind ourselves that we should respect all *perspectives* and avoid looking up only for this type of information that would support our own beliefs. In other words, we should avoid the so-called *"cherry-picking"* when choosing our sources of information and knowledge.

In this last chapter, we'll see how to distinguish true information from the one that could even be truer.

Avoid the "hook"

Indeed... how could we do that?

How can we learn to recognize when a certain bit of information is reliable and when it isn't?

How can we filter out the materials that would give us quality than the ones created with... other motives?

Even though it's not always so easy to apply these filters, the misinformation and disinformation still have some elements that aren't typical for the reliable, science-based information.

Here are some of them:

- **Information, inviting you to purchase a product**

If the text offers you to buy yet another "unique" organic food or an amazing supplement, then most probably we're talking about "adapting" the "facts" provided on purpose.

It's widely spread for all sorts of specialists, nutritionists and coaches to advertise certain supplements and products, and in almost all of the cases, the reasons behind that product recommendation are mainly commercial.

- **Information, promising fast results**

If the text *guarantees* that the product or service will have an immediate effect and the facts provided simply sound too good to be true, then most probably... they are *not* true.

Most of the time, promising fast and simple solutions to complex matters is simply an effective marketing trick for, guess what - making more money.

- **Information, causing fear**

We all have seen the following headlines:

*"Carbs make you **FAT!**"*

*"Artificial sweeteners are **TOXIC!**"*

*"Sugar – the white **DEATH!**"*

Having whole food groups removed from your menu due to similar statements also means depriving yourself of the nutrients that are found in these foods.

All this could lead to major food deficiencies, and anathematizing certain foods can cause serious eating disorders.

- **Information, defining what is "good" and "bad"**

Neither foods nor diets are good or bad on their own.

The problem is mainly hidden in the *quantity*.

"Bad" foods are often more calorie-dense and lack vitamins and minerals. Of course, they're tasty, so this could lead to higher quantities consumed without realizing it.

In fact, the "unhealthy" effect of such foods comes not from their presence in our diet, but because of the *absence* of the foods that could give our bodies the so vital micronutrients.

Therefore, the whole conception of categorizing foods as "good" and "bad" is wrong. And it's one of the main reasons for people to develop a bad relationship with them which, again, could lead to eating disorders.

So, that's why experts recommend that we talk about food as one that we can consume *often* and one that we can consume *from time to time*.

- **Information, entirely based on experience**

Okay, things here are simple – sharing an example from your own experience could often be useful for the others, but if there is nothing *evidence-based* that supports that information, this should ring the alarm for you.

- **Information based on just a few sources**

Very often you can spot a reading that seems to be well-structured at first glance, but if the cited references are only a few, then most probably the purpose of the text is only to support the sources mentioned and the author's statement.

In this way, you're not presented with the different points of view and the seemingly good information turns out to be misinforming.

- **Information based on studies with an irrelevant methodology**

We're talking here about all these texts that refer to dozens of scientific works, but the majority of them have no *direct* relation to the case in discussion.

For example, studies that have been conducted on animals or only in an in vitro environment. Or studies conducted on a non-randomized and a small group of people.

What do the complicated words mean?

Of course, talking about literature based on scientific evidence, we need to remember that the most important things are the *studies* themselves.

People often get confused about all the different types of scientific works. What do they all mean? Which ones are the most reliable?

Yes, the types are a lot but still, the main ones remain:

- **Expert opinions**

Honestly, they aren't qualified as sufficiently good evidence that could provide an answer to complex case studies because of their aptitude for prejudice and lack of systematic look and clear-cut set of criteria.

Still, they could be a decent *starting point* in the search for "truth" journey.

- **Systematic reviews**

They provide a response to a defined research question by collecting and summarizing all empiric pieces of evidence that have met certain predefined criteria.

Their purpose is the chance of errors made to be reduced to the minimum, thus providing a basis for more reliable findings, decisions, and conclusions.

- **Meta-analysis**

Simply said, this is a statistic technique for analyzing big, complex and even sometimes contradictory quantity of literature, the results of which are used for an assessment of previous studies.

Its benefit is that it allows the more accurate prediction of the effect of a given treatment or the risk factors of a given disease, compared to any other separate study that contributes to the analysis.

- **Randomized controlled studies**

They're considered the "*golden standard*" of the scientific practice for a reason.

Usually, they compare different results via random allocation of the participants in (most often) two groups. One of the groups (the test group) is given the tested substance, while the other (the control group) is presented with a placebo.

The advantage here is the *randomization* – it leads to a minimal number of mistakes that could be made out of a prejudiced attitude.

And yet, that type of study is far from perfect. They're often too expensive to conduct. Also, tested people cannot be classified as a cross-section of the whole population.

- **Cohort studies**

They're long-term observations on a group of people (called a *cohort*) that is exposed to supposedly risk factors with the sole purpose of detecting any changes in their health.

With time, a second group, that isn't exposed to the same conditions, is also observed.

The art of science

"Okay, okay... but why do we need all that?" Why do we need to trust science?", some might ask.

Probably you've heard how many scientists change their opinion very often – then how can we believe them, right?

To be honest, that observation is just somewhat true, as the true examples of scientists who had changed completely their perspective are only a few.

Indeed, sometimes they really do change their point of view while looking for new evidence – but, think about it - this is more *positive* than negative for science... and *us*. The changes in their opinion could potentially lead to the discovery of some new answers to old questions or discovering and investigating some new matters, even. This is how true *progress* has been made.

Through progress, science nowadays is much more than the well-known but outdated *"scientific method"* that tests with an experiment every new hypothesis.

Modern science is *dynamic* – nowadays, there are many improved methods that slowly but surely replace the old ones – and that process is constantly evolving with time.

Exactly over time, science has established that the considered by then ideally working "scientific method" was, in fact, a quite confusing tool as *wrong* theories could, accidentally or not, lead to... *accurate* results.

In other words, even if a given experiment works out, this doesn't mean that the theories that led to the whole experiment, are true. There are also cases when even completely *different* theories could lead to *similar* experiment results.

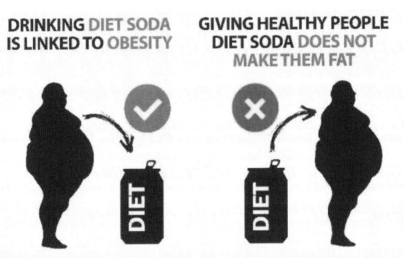

Correlation is not causality
Source: ebtofficial.com

And that's not all - if an experiment fails, does this mean that the theory is wrong, as well? Well, in some cases – yes, but in others... not really – the reason for the failure might simply be a bad design of the experiment or even incorrect reading of the results.

And since there is no perfect and universal scientific method, then how could we know what to trust and what not?

And the answer here is not to be found in the methods used by the scientists to generate statements, but in the methods that *assess* these statements.

No matter if we're talking about science related to climate changes or science related to food nutrients, the final statements of the scientists are always reviewed in all the tiny details and with the most critical eyes. And that is used to filter out the greater part of the wrong scientific statements so that at the end we have only those that have a much higher chance to prove correct.

And that filter is quite serious. For any scientific statement to be accepted and validated, it goes through a series of inspections, rules, procedures, and checks.

Of course, it all starts a bit informal – scientists first discuss the idea and its future design with each other and that discussion is eventually being transferred to conferences and seminars. It's a common thing for the design to get changed a few times, because of additional data gathering and more detailed revisions required.

After all that is done, qualified people are contacted for their feedback and if it's necessary, all is repeated multiple times, as much as necessary, till a final statement, supported by excellent examples, facts, analysis, and conclusion, is achieved.

And this is still not all.

In fact, this whole process is the easier part of the long journey a scientific statement takes before getting approved.

After the whole work is systemized, it's sent to a specific scientific journal to have it officially approved and then published to the wider community. The approval in question is obtained after a long and *extremely* demanding audit which aims at having even the slightest ambiguities and errors in the methodology and research sorted out.

If minor discrepancies are found, all the papers are sent back to the author(s) for correction. If corrections are necessary far too often or a major error is found in the papers, the journal has its right to simply cancel everything and to refuse to publish the work. And this is completely justified – after all, most of the scientific journals have a flawless reputation and they'd never risk their name by publishing studies that contain statements that might turn out to be unclear or even wrong.

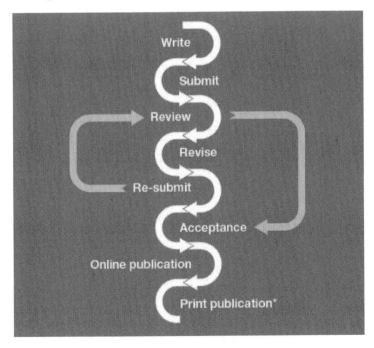

The process of true knowledge
Source: us.sagepub.com

A huge part of the references used in the book series is based on works published in the *top* scientific and medical journals. Of course, if you have carefully read the lines above, you'd understand that it's not reasonable to claim that *all* of them are accurate or could be considered the ultimate truth that should never be under the lash.

Yet, you see that the work of the scientists doesn't come to us that easily, it goes through many different channels to finally reach us in the form that we'd be sure in its correctness and conclusions.

Therefore, let the actors teach us how to play, let the singers teach us how to sing, let the mechanics give us advice about our car.

And let not anything else but *science* lead us to the true, evidence-based *knowledge*.

And let's use that knowledge to develop a culture of eating that's based not on the next "modern" diet, but on our sincere *preferences*. And thus, with fewer struggles and stress, with slower steps, and with more *pleasure*, to once and for all get that vision that we've always dreamt of.

Liked that? Let others know

If you enjoyed reading this book, it would be really appreciated if you spend about a minute or two and share your opinion.

Perhaps you think this doesn't matter that much but in reality, reviews are very helpful for me as an author.

They let me know what you have enjoyed in the content (or what you did not). And they could give me great ideas for potential future publications as well.

So, if you did enjoy this book and would like others to be able to discover it too, feel free to share your thoughts on it.

Thank you.

There's even more!

Seems like you really do trust verified information and evidence-based materials about healthy eating, don't you?

So, if you liked this book and want to learn more about the most popular undying food myths, (un)healthy practices, and beliefs, go get the first book of this series:

Enjoy Food!... and the top myths that still prevent you from doing so

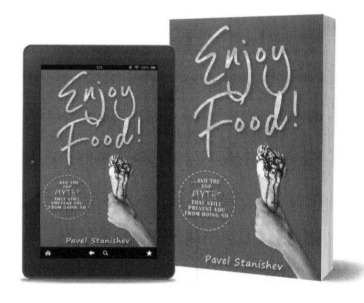

References

1. FoodData Central Search Results; *Bananas, raw*, U.S. Department of Agriculture – Agricultural Research Service; Accessed on 12 June 2019. Retrieved from: https://fdc.nal.usda.gov/fdc-app.html#/food-details/173944/nutrients

2. T P Wycherley, L J Moran, P M Clifton, M Noakes, G D Brinkworth; *Effects of energy-restricted high-protein, low-fat compared with standard-protein, low-fat diets: a meta-analysis of randomized controlled trials*, The American Journal of Clinical Nutrition, Volume 96, Issue 6, December 2012, Pages 1281–1298. Retrieved from: https://doi.org/10.3945/ajcn.112.044321

3. J W Krieger, H S Sitren, M J Daniels, B Langkamp-Henken; *Effects of variation in protein and carbohydrate intake on body mass and composition during energy restriction: a meta-regression*, The American Journal of Clinical Nutrition, Volume 83, Issue 2, February 2006, Pages 260–274. Retrieved from: https://doi.org/10.1093/ajcn/83.2.260

4. M S Westerterp-Plantenga, A Nieuwenhuizen, D Tomé, S Soenen, K R Westerterp; *Dietary Protein, Weight Loss, and Weight Maintenance*, Annual Review of Nutrition, Volume 29, Issue 1, August 2009, Pages 21-41. Retrieved from: https://doi.org/10.1146/annurev-nutr-080508-141056

5. K R Westerterp; *Nutrition & Metabolism: Diet induced thermogenesis*, Westerterp; licensee BioMed Central Ltd. 2004, Volume 1, Issue 1, August 2004, Page 1. Retrieved from: https://doi.org/10.1186/1743-7075-1-5

6. E Jéquier; *Pathways to obesity*, Springer Nature: International Journal of Obesity, Volume 26, Issue 2, August

2002, Pages S12-S17. Retrieved from:
https://doi.org/10.1038/sj.ijo.0802123

7. B A Magnuson, G A Burdock, J Doull, R M Kroes, G M
Marsh, M W Pariza, P S Spencer, W J Waddell, R Walker, G
M Williams; *Aspartame: A Safety Evaluation Based on
Current Use Levels, Regulations, and Toxicological and
Epidemiological Studies*, Critical Reviews In Toxicology
Journal, Volume 37, Issue 8, October 2008, Pages 629-727.
Retrieved from:
https://doi.org/10.1080/10408440701516184

8. DrugBank; *Aspartame*, DrugBank.ca; Accessed on 21 June
2019. Retrieved from:
https://www.drugbank.ca/drugs/DB00168

9. M Franz MS, RD, LD; *AMOUNTS OF SWEETENERS IN
POPULAR DIET SODAS*, Diabetes Self-Management, R.A.
Rapaport Publishing, Inc.; Accessed on 21 June 2019.
Retrieved from:
http://static.diabetesselfmanagement.com/pdfs/DSM0310
012.pdf

10. D Whitbread, MScN; *Top 10 Foods Highest in
Phenylalanine*, MyFoodData.com; April 2019; Accessed on
21 June 2019. Retrieved from:
https://www.myfooddata.com/articles/high-phenylalanine-
foods.php

11. U.S. Food & Drug Administration; *Additional Information
about High-Intensity Sweeteners Permitted for Use in Food
in the United States*, FDA.gov, August 2018; Accessed on 21
June 2019. Retrieved from: https://www.fda.gov/food/food-
additives-petitions/additional-information-about-high-
intensity-sweeteners-permitted-use-food-united-
states#Aspartame

12. European Food Safety Authority; Aspartame,
EFSA.Europa.eu; Accessed on 21 June 2019. Retrieved from:
https://www.efsa.europa.eu/en/topics/topic/aspartame

13. World Health Organization; *ASPARTAME*, Evaluations of the Joint FAO/WHO Expert Committee on Food Additives (JECFA); Accessed on 21 June 2019. Retrieved from: http://apps.who.int/food-additives-contaminants-jecfa-database/chemical.aspx?chemID=62

14. H H Butchko, F N Kotsonis; *Acceptable daily intake vs actual intake: the aspartame example.*, Journal of the American College of Nutrition, Volume 10, Issue 3, June 1991, Pages 258-266. Retrieved from: https://www.ncbi.nlm.nih.gov/pubmed/1894884

15. National Organization for Rare Disorders; Phenylketonuria, RareDiseases.org; Accessed on 21 June 2019. Retrieved from: https://rarediseases.org/rare-diseases/phenylketonuria/

16. U.S. Environmental Protection Agency; *Toxicological Review of Methanol (Noncancer) (CAS No. 67-56-1) In Support of Summary Information on the Integrated Risk Information System (IRIS)*, epa.gov/iris, September 2013, EPA/635/R-11/001Fa; Retrieved from: https://cfpub.epa.gov/ncea/iris/iris_documents/documents/toxreviews/0305tr.pdf

17. European Food Safety Authority; *Scientific Opinion on Aspartame*, EFSA.Europa.eu; Accessed on 21 June 2019. Retrieved from: https://www.efsa.europa.eu/sites/default/files/corporate_publications/files/factsheetaspartame.pdf

18. S S Schiffman, Ph.D., C E Buckley, III, M.D., H A Sampson, M.D., E W Massey, M.D., J N Baraniuk, M.D., J V Follett, M.D., Z S Warwick, B.S; *Aspartame and Susceptibility to Headache*, The New England Journal of Medicine, Volume 317, Issue 19, November 1987, Pages 1181-1185. Retrieved from: https://doi.org/10.1056/NEJM198711053171903

19. K A Lapierre M.D., D J Greenblatt M.D., J E Goddard M.A., J S Harmatz B.A., R I Shader M.D.; *The Neuropsychiatric*

Effects of Aspartame in Normal Volunteers, The Journal of Clinical Pharmacology, Volume 30, Issue 5, May 1990, Pages 454-460. Retrieved from: https://doi.org/10.1002/j.1552-4604.1990.tb03485.x

20. R Geha M.D., C E Buckley M.D., P Greenberger M.D., R Patterson M.D., S Polmar M.D., PhD, A Saxon M.D., A Rohr M.D., W Yang M.D., M Drouin M.D.; *Aspartame is no more likely than placebo to cause urticaria/angioedema: Results of a multicenter, randomized, double-blind, placebo-controlled, crossover study*, The Journal of Allergy and Clinical Immunology, Volume 92, Issue 4, October 1993, Pages 513-520. Retrieved from: https://www.jacionline.org/article/0091-6749(93)90075-Q/fulltext

21. M Vellisca, J I Latorre; *Monosodium glutamate and aspartame in perceived pain in fibromyalgia*, Rheumatology International, Volume 34, Issue 7, July 2014, Pages 1011-1013. Retrieved from: https://doi.org/10.1007/s00296-013-2801-5

22. Dr. B A Shaywitz M.D., G M Anderson PhD, E J Novotny M.D., J S Ebersole M.D., C M Sullivan MSN, S M Gillespie MSN; *Aspartame has no effect on seizures or epileptiform discharges in epileptic children*, Annals of Neurology – An Official Journal of the American Neurological Association and the Child Neurology Society, Volume 35, Issue 1, January 1994, Pages 98-103. Retrieved from: https://doi.org/10.1002/ana.410350115

23. A J Rowan, B A Shaywitz, L Tuchman, J A French, D Luciano, C M Sullivan; *Aspartame and Seizure Susceptibility: Results of a Clinical Study in Reportedly Sensitive Individuals*, Epilepsia, Official Journal of the International League Against Epilepsy, Volume 36, Issue 3, March 1995, Pages 270-275. Retrieved from: https://doi.org/10.1111/j.1528-1157.1995.tb00995.x

24. M Soffritti, F Belpoggi, D D Esposti, L Lambertini; *Aspartame induces lymphomas and leukaemias in rats*, European Journal of Oncology, Volume 10, Issue 2, June 2005, Pages 107-116. Retrieved from: https://www.researchgate.net/publication/225029050_Asp artame_induces_lymphomas_and_leukaemias_in_rats

25. National Cancer Institute; *Artificial Sweeteners and Cancer*; National Institutes of Health, Cancer.org, August 2016; Accessed on 21 June 2019. Retrieved from: https://www.cancer.gov/about-cancer/causes-prevention/risk/diet/artificial-sweeteners-fact-sheet#r2

26. National Toxicology Program; *NTP report on the toxicology studies of aspartame (CAS No. 22839-47-0) in genetically modified (FVB Tg.AC hemizygous) and B6.129-Cdkn2atm1Rdp (N2) deficient mice and carcinogenicity studies of aspartame in genetically modified [B6.129-Trp53tm1Brd (N5) haploinsufficient] mice (feed studies).*, U.S. Department of Health and Human Services, Volume 1, October 2005, Pages 1-222. Retrieved from: https://www.ncbi.nlm.nih.gov/pubmed/18685711

27. European Food Safety Authority; *EFSA assesses new aspartame study and reconfirms its safety*, EFSA.Europa.eu, May 2006; Accessed on 21 June 2019. Retrieved from: https://www.efsa.europa.eu/en/press/news/060504

28. U Lim, A F Subar, T Mouw, P Hartge, L M Morton, R Stolzenberg-Solomon, D Campbell, A R Hollenbeck, A Schatzkin; *Consumption of Aspartame-Containing Beverages and Incidence of Hematopoietic and Brain Malignancies*, Cancer Epidemiology, Biomarkers & Prevention, Volume 15, Issue 9, September 2006, Pages 1654-1659. Retrieved from: https://doi.org/10.1158/1055-9965.EPI-06-0203

29. M Marinovich, C L Galli, C Bosetti, S Gallus, C La Vecchia; *Aspartame, low-calorie sweeteners and disease: Regulatory safety and epidemiological issues*, Food and Chemical Toxicology, Volume 60, October 2013, Pages 109-115. Retrieved from: https://doi.org/10.1016/j.fct.2013.07.040

30. T Sathyapalan, N J Thatcher, R Hammersley, A S Rigby, A Pechlivanis, N J Gooderham, E Holmes, C W le Roux, S L Atkin, F Courts; *Aspartame Sensitivity? A Double Blind Randomised Crossover Study*, Public Library of Science, Volume 10, Issue 3, March 2015. Retrieved from: https://doi.org/10.1371/journal.pone.0116212

31. Q Yang; *Gain weight by "going diet?" Artificial sweeteners and the neurobiology of sugar cravings: Neuroscience 2010*, The Yale Journal of Biology and Medicine, Volume 83, Issue 2, June 2010, Pages 101-108. Retrieved from: https://www.ncbi.nlm.nih.gov/pmc/articles/PMC2892765/

32. New York Academy of Medicine Library; *The United Fruit Company's Food Value of the Banana, ca. 1928.*, November 2015. Retrieved from: https://library.nyam.org/2unitedfruitcompany_foodvaluebanana_1928_cover/

33. SELFNutritionData; *Bananas, raw Nutrition Facts & Calories*. Retrieved from: https://nutritiondata.self.com/facts/fruits-and-fruit-juices/1846/2

34. Google Trends; *Search term "goji berry"*. Accessed on 2 August 2019. Retrieved from: https://trends.google.com/trends/explore?date=all&q=goji%20berry

35. R J Williams, J P E Spencer, C Rice-Evans; *Flavonoids: antioxidants or signalling molecules?*, Free Radical Biology and Medicine, Volume 36, Issue 7, April 2004, Pages 838-

849. Retrieved from:
https://doi.org/10.1016/j.freeradbiomed.2004.01.001

36. S B Lotito, B Frei; *Consumption of flavonoid-rich foods and increased plasma antioxidant capacity in humans: Cause, consequence, or epiphenomenon?*, Free Radical Biology and Medicine, Volume 41, Issue 12, December 2006, Pages 1727-1746. Retrieved from:
https://doi.org/10.1016/j.freeradbiomed.2006.04.033

37. SELFNutritionData; *Blueberries, raw Nutrition Facts & Calories*. Retrieved from:
https://nutritiondata.self.com/facts/fruits-and-fruit-juices/1851/2

38. SELFNutritionData; *Raspberries, raw Nutrition Facts & Calories*. Retrieved from:
https://nutritiondata.self.com/facts/fruits-and-fruit-juices/2053/2

39. SELFNutritionData; *Blackberries, raw Nutrition Facts & Calories*. Retrieved from:
https://nutritiondata.self.com/facts/fruits-and-fruit-juices/1848/2

40. SELFNutritionData; *Avocados, raw, all commercial varieties Nutrition Facts & Calories*. Retrieved from:
https://nutritiondata.self.com/facts/fruits-and-fruit-juices/1843/2

41. S Wagner, H Breiteneder; *The latex-fruit syndrome*, Biochemical Society Transactions, Volume 30, Issue 6, November 2002, Pages 935-940. Retrieved from:
https://doi.org/10.1042/bst0300935

42. D Pendick; *Can't touch this: "Latex-free" labels are misleading*, Harvard Health Publishing, March 2013. Retrieved from: https://www.health.harvard.edu/blog/cant-touch-this-latex-free-labels-are-misleading-201303135973

43. SELFNutritionData; *Quinoa, cooked Nutrition Facts & Calories*. Retrieved from:

https://nutritiondata.self.com/facts/cereal-grains-and-pasta/10352/2

44. SELFNutritionData; *Beans, kidney, all types, mature seeds, cooked, boiled, without salt Nutrition Facts & Calories.* Retrieved from: https://nutritiondata.self.com/facts/legumes-and-legume-products/4297/2

45. ScienceDirect; *Phytic Acid*, ScienceDirect.com. Retrieved from: https://www.sciencedirect.com/topics/agricultural-and-biological-sciences/phytic-acid

46. S Sivapalan; *Nutritional aspects of quinoa*, Department of Primary Industries and Regional Development's Agriculture and Food, Government of Western Australia, October 2018. Retrieved from: https://www.agric.wa.gov.au/irrigated-crops/nutritional-aspects-quinoa

47. R Nagel; *Living With Phytic Acid*, The Weston A. Price Foundation, March 2010. Retrieved from: https://www.westonaprice.org/health-topics/vegetarianism-and-plant-foods/living-with-phytic-acid/

48. Tridge; *Quinoa*, Tridge.com. Accessed on 24 July 2019. Retrieved from: https://www.tridge.com/intelligences/quinoa

49. Tridge; *Rice*, Tridge.com. Accessed on 24 July 2019. Retrieved from: https://www.tridge.com/intelligences/rice

50. Tridge; *Maize (Corn)*, Tridge.com. Accessed on 24 July 2019. Retrieved from: https://www.tridge.com/intelligences/corn

51. Tridge; *Millet*, Tridge.com. Accessed on 24 July 2019. Retrieved from: https://www.tridge.com/intelligences/millet

52. A L Reuterswärd; *The new EC Regulation on nutrition and health claims on foods*, Scandinavian Journal of Food & Nutrition, Volume 51, Issue 3, 2007, Pages 100-106.

Retrieved from:
https://www.ncbi.nlm.nih.gov/pmc/articles/PMC2606979/?report=reader

53. SELFNutritionData; *Chicken, liver, all classes, cooked, simmered Nutrition Facts & Calories.* Retrieved from: https://nutritiondata.self.com/facts/poultry-products/667/2

54. M Chaplin; *Water: A Brief Early History of its Science,* Water Structure and Science, May 2019. Retrieved from: http://www1.lsbu.ac.uk/water/water.html

55. H Valtin; *"Drink at least eight glasses of water a day." Really? Is there scientific evidence for "8 x 8"?*, The American Physiology Society, Volume 283, Issue 5, November 2002, Pages R993-1004. Retrieved from: https://doi.org/10.1152/ajpregu.00365.2002

56. J Murphy; *8 glasses of water a day: Myth or medicine?*, MDLinx, October 2018. Retrieved from: https://bit.ly/2Z3oXwT

57. J S Berns MD, S Goldfarb MD; *Drinking Water: What's the Science?*, Medscape.com, WebMD LLC, June 2014. Retrieved from: https://www.medscape.com/viewarticle/826504

58. B M Popkin, K E D'Anci, I H Rosenberg; Water, Hydration and Health, Nutrition Reviews, Volume 68, Issue 8, August 2010, Pages 439-458. Retrieved from: https://doi.org/10.1111/j.1753-4887.2010.00304.x

59. Institute of Medicine of the National Academies; *Dietary Reference Intakes for Water, Potassium, Sodium, Chloride, and Sulfate,* The National Academies Press, February 2004. Retrieved from: http://www.nationalacademies.org/hmd/Reports/2004/Dietary-Reference-Intakes-Water-Potassium-Sodium-Chloride-and-Sulfate.aspx

60. Google Trends; *Search term "lemon water"*. Accessed on 14 November 2019. Retrieved from: https://trends.google.com/trends/explore?date=all&q=lemon%20water

61. S N Kreitzman, A Y Coxon, K F Szaz; *Glycogen storage: illusions of easy weight loss, excessive weight regain, and distortions in estimates of body composition*, The American Journal of Clinical Nutrition, Volume 56, Issue 1, July 1992, Pages 292S–293S. Retrieved from: https://doi.org/10.1093/ajcn/56.1.292S

62. H M Parretti, P Aveyard, A Blannin, S J Clifford, S J Coleman, A Roalfe, A J Daley; *Efficacy of water preloading before main meals as a strategy for weight loss in primary care patients with obesity: RCT*, Obesity: A Research Journal, The Obesity Society, Volume 23, Issue 9, September 2015, Pages 1785-1791. Retrieved from: https://doi.org/10.1002/oby.21167

63. B M Davy PhD RD, E A Dennis, A L Dengo MS, K L Wilson, K P Davy PhD; *Water Consumption Reduces Energy Intake at a Breakfast Meal in Obese Older Adults, Journal of the American Dietetic Association*, Volume 108, Issue 7, July 2008, Pages 1236-1239. Retrieved from: https://doi.org/10.1016/j.jada.2008.04.013

64. E L Van Walleghen, J S Orr, C L Gentile, B M Davy; *Pre-meal Water Consumption Reduces Meal Energy Intake in Older but Not Younger Subjects*, Obesity: A Research Journal, The Obesity Society, Volume 15, Issue 1, January 2007, Pages 93-99. Retrieved from: https://doi.org/10.1038/oby.2007.506

65. E A Dennis, A L Dengo, D L Comber, K D Flack, J Savla, K P Davy, B M Davy; *Water Consumption Increases Weight Loss During a Hypocaloric Diet Intervention in Middle-aged and Older Adults*, Obesity: A Research Journal, The Obesity Society, Volume 18, Issue 2, February 2010, Pages

300-307. Retrieved from:
https://doi.org/10.1038/oby.2009.235

66. M M Reicks, D Crankshaw; *Effects of D-limonene on hepatic microsomal monooxygenase activity and paracetamol-induced glutathione depletion in mouse*, Xenobiotica: the fate of foreign compounds in biological systems, Volume 23, Issue 7, Mar 1993, Pages 809-817. Retrieved from:
https://doi.org/10.3109/00498259309166786

67. The Free Dictionary by Farlex; *Search term "pH scale"*, Farlex Inc. Accessed on 14 November 2019. Retrieved from:
https://medical-dictionary.thefreedictionary.com/pH+scale

68. L L Hamm, N Nakhoul, K S Hering-Smith; *Acid-Base Homeostasis*, Clinical Journal of American Society of Nephrology, Volume 10, Issue 12, December 2015, Pages 2232-2242. Retrieved from:
https://doi.org/10.2215/CJN.07400715

69. J Leech MS; *The Alkaline Diet: An Evidence-Based Review*, Healthline Media, September 2019. Retrieved from:
https://www.healthline.com/nutrition/the-alkaline-diet-myth#impact-of-food

70. Google Trends; *Search term "raw water"*. Accessed on 14 November 2019. Retrieved from:
https://trends.google.com/trends/explore?date=all&q=%2F m%2F04g7cg

71. K Zeratsky RD LD; *I've heard friends talk about switching to raw water. Why is this so popular?*, Mayo Clinic, May 2019. Retrieved from: https://www.mayoclinic.org/healthy-lifestyle/nutrition-and-healthy-eating/expert-answers/raw-water/faq-20406843

72. R Fisher, L Malmud, P Bandini, E Rock; *Gastric Emptying of a Physiologic Mixed Solid-Liquid Meal*, Clinical Nuclear Medicine, Volume 7, Issue 5, May 1982, Pages 215-221. Retrieved from: https://doi.org/10.1097/00003072-198205000-00005

73. ScienceDirect.com; *Stomach Secretion*, Elsevier B.V. Retrieved from: https://www.sciencedirect.com/topics/medicine-and-dentistry/stomach-secretion

74. E A Dennis, A L Dengo, D L Comber, K D Flack, J Savla, K P Davy, B M Davy; *Water Consumption Increases Weight Loss During a Hypocaloric Diet Intervention in Middle-aged and Older Adults*, Obesity: A Research Journal, The Obesity Society, Volume 18, Issue 2, February 2010, Pages 300-307. Retrieved from: https://doi.org/10.1038/oby.2009.235

Printed in Great Britain
by Amazon